Reflective Teaching & Learning in the Health Professions

Action Research in Professional Education

Reflective Teaching & Learning in the Health Professions

Action Research in Professional Education

David Kember

with

Alice Jones, Alice Yuen Loke, Jan McKay
Kit Sinclair, Harrison Tse, Celia Webb
Frances Kam Yuet Wong, Marian Wai Lin Wong and Ella Yeung

Blackwell
Science

© 2001 by
Blackwell Science Ltd
Editorial Offices:
Osney Mead, Oxford OX2 0EL
25 John Street, London WC1N 2BS
23 Ainslie Place, Edinburgh EH3 6AJ
350 Main Street, Malden
    MA 02148 5018, USA
54 University Street, Carlton
    Victoria 3053, Australia
10, rue Casimir Delavigne
    75006 Paris, France

Other Editorial Offices:

Blackwell Wissenschafts-Verlag GmbH
Kurfürstendamm 57
10707 Berlin, Germany

Blackwell Science KK
MG Kodenmacho Building
7–10 Kodenmacho Nihombashi
Chuo-ku, Tokyo 104, Japan

Iowa State University Press
A Blackwell Science Company
2121 S. State Avenue
Ames, Iowa 50014-8300, USA

The right of the Author to be identified as
the Author of this Work has been asserted in
accordance with the Copyright, Designs and
Patents Act 1988.

First published 2001

Set in 11/12 Sabon
by DP Photosetting, Aylesbury, Bucks
Printed and bound in Great Britain by
MPG Books Ltd, Bodmin, Cornwall

The Blackwell Science logo is a trade mark of
Blackwell Science Ltd, registered at the
United Kingdom Trade Marks Registry

DISTRIBUTORS

Marston Book Services Ltd
PO Box 269
Abingdon
Oxon OX14 4YN
(*Orders*:   Tel: 01235 465500
             Fax: 01235 465555)

USA
Blackwell Science, Inc.
Commerce Place
350 Main Street
Malden, MA 02148 5018
(*Orders*:   Tel: 800 759 6102
                  781 388 8250
             Fax: 781 388 8250)

Canada
Login Brothers Book Company
324 Saulteaux Crescent
Winnipeg, Manitoba R3J 3T2
(*Orders*:   Tel: 204 837-2987
             Fax: 204 837-3116)

Australia
Blackwell Science Pty Ltd
54 University Street
Carlton, Victoria 3053
(*Orders*:   Tel: 03 9347 0300
             Fax: 03 9347 5001)

A catalogue record for this title is available
from the British Library

ISBN 0-632-05739-4

Library of Congress
Cataloging-in-Publication Data
    Reflective teaching and learning in the
health professions: action research in
professional education/David Kember
        p.   cm
    Includes bibliographical references and
index.
    ISBN 0-632-05739-4
    1. Medicine–Study and teaching.
2. Thought and thinking.   3. Medical
education.   4. Learning
I. Kember, David.
R737.R344 2000
610'71'1–dc21
                                    00-052963

For further information on
Blackwell Science, visit our website:
www.blackwell-science.com

Contents

Preface

What this book is about

The aim of this book is to enable students in the health professions to fully combine the theory aspect of their courses with the professional practice element by encouraging them to adopt reflective practice.

Many students find the task of applying theory taught in the classroom to the reality of professional practice extremely difficult until they develop the ability to reflect on the relationship between the two.

The concept of reflection continues to excite considerable interest among professional educators, and the question of how best to design and implement courses which encourage reflection remains much-discussed but hitherto unresolved. There are also more theoretical concerns over the interpretation of the reflective process as well as the distinction between reflective and non-reflective action. This book was prompted by a project which attempted to address these issues and provide some answers to the questions below.

The questions which follow are inter-related. The first four were tackled through an action research approach. Cycles of planning, action, observation and reflection were used to test and refine components which had been designed to promote reflection in five professional courses for health care workers. The five courses were examined simultaneously which made comparison possible, and allowed lessons learnt from one to be applied to others. Conclusions about reflective teaching were synthesised from this research.

Evaluating the five courses resulted in a lot of mainly qualitative data derived from reflective journals, interviews and classroom observation. These data were then used to try and answer the following questions and associated subquestions.

How can courses be designed to encourage reflective thinking?

How should a course be formulated if it is to promote reflection-in-action and reflection on reflection-in-action? The use of student diaries, reports, learning contracts, discussion sessions and regular disclosures was investigated. The problematic issues of assessment and the teacher's access to students' reflective writing were examined.

How can obstacles to reflective thinking be overcome?

What are the factors that prevent students from engaging successfully in reflective practice? How can they be overcome? Do some students find it harder than others to become reflective? In order to construct an ideal learning environment for reflectivity, what educational factors – class size, workload, course structure and assessment methods – should be taken into account?

How can theory and practice best be integrated in professional courses?

Reflective practice is often advocated as a means of bridging the gap between the theory and practice parts of professional courses. However it is unclear whether this is successful when students are asked to be reflective only in the practice parts of their courses. It is also doubtful that students will reflect upon their practice if they have not developed appropriate conceptions of knowledge and reflective judgement. This book explains how to integrate theory and practice by developing reflective practice in both parts of professional courses.

How can students' reflective practice be assessed?

It is impossible to know whether the aims of a course designed to promote reflective thinking have been achieved unless some form of assessment is involved. A suitable form of assessment is not easy to design, however. There appear to be few accepted procedures to assess the level of reflective thinking that a student has achieved, and the very act of assessing reflective writing can discourage the personal introspection which the course is designed to encourage. On the other hand, students do not always afford the same respect to courses which they know are not going to be assessed. During the research work carried out on the project behind this book several balanced positions were achieved which appeared to offer a compromise. A procedure for assessing the level of reflection in written journals was developed (Kember, Jones, Loke, McKay, Sinclair, Tse, Webb, Wong, Wong & Yeung, 1999), and a questionnaire to measure the levels of reflection the students were achieving (Kember, Leung, Jones, Loke, McKay, Sinclair, Tse, Webb, Wong, Wong & Yeung, in press). These are reported in detail elsewhere.

Are existing models of reflection adequate?

Our review of the existing literature on reflection revealed writings which had emanated from particular academic traditions and were applied to specific contexts. However, there was often little cross-referencing between these literature categories. As a result the same terms could be used to mean quite different things by different writers, and descriptions of reflective thinking processes could have narrow, context-bound frames of reference. Since this book is intended to cross the theory/practice divide, one aim has been to establish a more general reflection language by drawing on the existing traditions.

The concept of reflection was also examined more empirically by analysing reflective writing, transcripts of interviews with students, and class discussions. These examinations were conducted from the perspective of the students' interpretation of the concept of reflection, and of how they employed reflective thinking in their clinical practice. As many of the students were already practising professionals who were studying part-time, they had current experience of professional and clinical practice upon which to draw.

David Kember

Acknowledgements

We wish to acknowledge all the students who have taken part in the various learning situations discussed in this book, and in particular those who have taken the time to contribute to the various feedback activities. The insight gained into the point of view of the learner has been invaluable.

We are grateful to Sally Candlin for her meticulous copy editing. We would also like to thank two reviewers for some very constructive comments upon an early draft: Chris Bulman from the School of Health Care, Oxford Brookes University, and Susan Ryan of the Department of Health Sciences, University of East London.

The project and the various sub-projects which led to this book were supported by grants from the University Grants Committee of Hong Kong, the Action Learning Project and the Hong Kong Polytechnic University.

Contributors

Alice Jones is an Associate Professor in Physiotherapy at the Department of Rehabilitation Sciences, The Hong Kong Polytechnic University. Her research interest is in cardio-pulmonary physiotherapy care as well as student learning. Her MSc was in the Practice of Higher Education from the University of Surrey, UK.

David Kember was the coordinator of the Action Learning Project when the project on which this book is based was carried out. The Action Learning Project was an inter-institutional initiative which supported academics in all eight universities in Hong Kong to conduct 90 action research projects into some aspect of courses they taught. David Kember is currently the Associate Director of Educational Development in the Hong Kong Polytechnic University; he has worked in a variety of educational development positions in the UK, Fiji, Papua New Guinea and Australia.

Alice Yuen Loke is an Associate Professor in Nursing in the Department of Nursing and Health Sciences. She received her Master's degree in Nursing Education and Community Health in 1985 from the United States, and her PhD from the Department of Community Medicine at the University of Hong Kong. She has been teaching at the Baccalaureate and Master's levels in nursing at universities in the United States and in Hong Kong since 1985. She is interested in nursing education as well as women's health.

Jan McKay is an Associate Professor in the Department of Optometry and Radiography. She leads the undergraduate radiography programme and chairs the department's Learning and Teaching Committee. In both roles she sees providing support and encouragement to further develop a student-centred learning philosophy as an important part of her brief.

Kit Sinclair is an Assistant Professor in Occupational Therapy in the Department of Rehabilitation Sciences. Her particular interest is reflective teaching and learning. An Honorary Fellow of the World Federation of Occupational Therapists, she has contributed significantly to the international promotion and development of occupational therapy, and provides regular consultancy to professional associations and education programmes worldwide. Her doctoral study is in the development of clinical reasoning in the academic arena.

Harrison Tse was the research fellow for the project on which this book is based. He was responsible for collecting and analysing qualitative and quantitative data obtained from observations, interviews and questionnaires. Besides being an active participant of the project, he was also a co-ordinator between project members. Harrison is currently a PhD candidate at the University of Newcastle upon Tyne.

After many years as a physiotherapist and clinical educator for student physiotherapists, **Celia Webb** completed a post-graduate course at the Institute of Education, London University, and the UK Chartered Society of Physiotherapy's Diploma Course for Teachers. She then taught at the School of Physiotherapy, Guys' Hospital, London, and later in the Department of Rehabilitation Sciences at the Hong Kong Polytechnic University, where she has been an associate professor. She co-ordinated clinical studies for physiotherapy students for several years and is very interested in progressing student learning, particularly in clinical, community and school settings.

Frances Kam Yuet Wong is an Associate Professor in Nursing in the Department of Nursing and Health Sciences. She has published widely in the areas of nursing education and contemporary nursing trends and development.

Marian Wai Lin Wong is an Assistant Professor in Nursing in the Department of Nursing and Health Sciences in Hong Kong Polytechnic University. She is a trained nurse, midwife and nurse educator. Her doctoral study is focused on understanding students' conceptualisation of nursing knowledge and the application of the conceptualisation to real-life nursing setting. Marian is very involved in the design, administration and delivery of various nursing programmes to meet service needs. She has a wide range of interests in nursing education and clinical nursing research.

Ella Yeung is an Assistant Professor in Physiotherapy at the Department of Rehabilitation Sciences, The Hong Kong Polytechnic University. Her interest in educational research involves students' learning process and outcome in problem-based learning. She has obtained two research grants to develop and implement this teaching methodology in the curriculum.

Preview

This section gives a brief preview of each part and chapter to help readers understand the structure of the book and the relationship of each part to the whole.

Part I: Introduction

The first part of the book introduces the concepts of reflection and reflective thinking. It also explains the project on which the book is based and the research methodology used for the study.

Chapter 1: The nature of reflection

The nature of professional practice is discussed, leading to the conclusion that professionals deal with ill-defined issues. Reflection-on-practice is then introduced as a means by which professionals deal with these 'messy' problems. The inference is drawn that professional education courses need to develop their students as reflective practitioners if they are to prepare them properly for their future careers. It is argued that the development of reflective thinking should be an integral component of the theory part of professional programmes and not confined to the period of professional practice, otherwise there will be no integration of theory and practice and students will not be equipped for their practice sessions.

In order to discuss the nature of reflection, the work of several prominent writers is examined. The conclusion is that a number of quite discrete areas of literature have developed according to the context of the work, and the tradition and discipline on which the writer is drawing.

Dewey (1933) wrote of reflective thinking as a thought process which education should strive to cultivate. King &

Kitchener (1994) argue that reflective judgement is a quality college students need to develop in order to recognise and deal with ill-defined problems. Schön's (1983) influential work is about professional practice and describes the reflective practices employed by professionals in a number of fields. Schön's (1987) work on educating professionals for reflective practice has been highly influential in the field of professional education in health sciences but needs adaptation and development because the studio education model it features is quite different from most professional education in health sciences.

Several writers in the field of adult education, most notably Mezirow (1981, 1991 and 1992), have derived categorical descriptions of reflection from critical theory. Others with backgrounds in adult education, such as Boud (1985; 1981) and Jarvis (1987, 1992, 1995), have taken a more experiential approach to propose models of reflective thinking processes. As this book integrates college-based education with professional practice, the authors felt it necessary to draw upon each of these contextually defined treatments of reflection and attempt a synthesised definition.

Chapter 2: Action research and its application to the project

The material on which this book is based is drawn from five, initially independent, action research projects into various aspects of reflective teaching. Bringing together the five strands facilitated reflection upon experiences and lessons learnt in each of the courses. The collective reflection made it possible to synthesise conclusions which were both more profound and more likely to be generally applicable. This chapter describes this approach of synthesising conclusions from multiple action research projects.

It also describes the process of analysing the large volume of data, initially gathered as part of the evaluation phase of the five course-based projects. The management and use of the database with NUD•IST software is detailed.

The chapter also deals with the context of education of health professionals in Hong Kong and makes comparison with international trends. It gives a brief description of the five courses so that the context of the project can be understood.

Part II: Developing reflective teaching in five healthcare courses

Part II presents the findings from the programme-level action research studies about specific topics in promoting reflection.

Chapter 3: The action research process

This chapter discusses the experience of promoting reflective practitioners through the action research approach using the nursing course as an example. The principles generated from the action research approach can be applied across different settings in educating healthcare professionals. The teaching team had a teaching initiative that they wanted to put into practice. Action research was found to be a useful strategy to help the team experiment with the new approach and make modifications throughout the process as they identified problems. Both teachers and students in action research are researchers and reflective practitioners. They regularly collect evidence, reflect on it and make modifications to guide their subsequent actions to maximise students' learning.

Chapter 4: Integrating theory and practice

This chapter discusses two initiatives that were taken to support a newly introduced programme which aimed to encourage student-centred learning by developing a reflective learning approach. In taking this approach there was a conscious effort made to move away from a previous technical-rational format used on the previous programme.

Both initiatives were aimed at encouraging students to be reflective about the theory they were learning, in the light of clinical experience, and addressed the problem of how to best encourage and support integration of theoretical learning with clinical practice.

Four cycles of action were completed with progressive developments being noted. There is a discussion of how the intervention influenced teaching and learning initiatives within the programme.

Chapter 5: The use of learning contracts

In the physiotherapy undergraduate programme, adoption of the learning contract approach was introduced to students and clinical educators to encourage reflection. As part of an action-learning programme, a number of students and their clinical educators participated in the evaluation of the learning process. Throughout the clinical placement, the students, the clinical educator and the lecturer concerned met once a week to discuss and evaluate the progress of the student. The aims were to identify strategies to facilitate the development of critical reflection in the student, to promote their ability in the synthesis of new ideas, to explore assumptions and then to think of alternative solutions and to generate conclusions. A more flexible approach to the implementation of learning contracts was found to assist with the development of more independent, in-depth and reflective learning for the students and the educator. There is a shift of focus from simply fulfilling objectives in the learning contract towards establishing a stronger relationship between the educators and the students.

Chapter 6: Writing reflective journals

First year undergraduate students were introduced to reflection early in their programme by requiring them to write reflective journal entries about specifically designed learning activities and clinical visit observations. In their journals, they were asked to explain their learning experience in their own words and relate it to their own past experience. Students were encouraged to use their journals to monitor their own progress and prepare for the assignment and final examination. They used their journals as a basis for contribution to group discussion and to share new ideas, problems and issues.

Students expressed concern about their lack of confidence in journal writing, noting an uncertainty about the staff expectations for journal writing, the contrast between experiential and classroom learning (the first being easier to write about), and difficulties of language style and expression. They also expressed a need for more group discussion.

In a second cycle of teaching, more specific guidelines on journal writing were provided to students with examples of previous students' work and more discussion time being provided throughout the course. Journal entries were collected and immediate written feedback was given. Students in the second cycle showed a better understanding of the overall aim of journal writing as a tool to learn and organise knowledge from their own experience. They appeared to take more initiative in writing about activities and feelings. They regarded the journal writing process as an opportunity for self-evaluation.

Chapter 7: Promoting discussion from reflective writing

In an attempt to introduce reflective concepts to clinical educators in an experiential manner, journal writing and reflective class discussion were made an integral part of a 14 week module on teaching and learning. Participants were asked to keep a reflective journal, to write about a subject of interest from their reading or from daily work experiences which was relevant to clinical education and the topics covered in the syllabus. They were asked to prepare one item from the journal to share in class discussion the following week.

Though some participants were initially unsure and frustrated by the perceived lack of guidelines for the reflective sessions, they spoke up regularly in class and had obviously prepared for the sessions. Class reflection seemed to reinforce their interest in their own reflective activity.

Journal reading and discussion provided the facilitators with the opportunity to monitor progress on the course and was a measure of where the students were in their understanding of various aspects of the material being covered relevant to clinical education. Feedback provided in this way meant that course material could be supplemented, discarded or changed to suit the needs of the students.

Part III: Synthesising conclusions about curricula

Part III presents the conclusions of the higher-level action research study of how to teach and design curricula which encourage students to engage in reflection upon their practice. These chapters present the conclusions synthesised from the five studies reported in Part II. The conclusions draw upon at least two courses in each case, and often all five courses.

Chapter 8: Encouraging reflective writing

How should courses be arranged if students are to be encouraged to reflect upon their practice through the writing of reflective journals? It was discovered that students needed an introduction to, and feedback on, reflective writing as it differed from other types of writing required in academic courses. For reflective writing to be taken seriously, it needed to be an integral part of the course. Issues such as the disclosure of journal entries and the assessment of reflective writing needed to be handled sensitively. The courses studied evolved positions on these issues which attempted to balance conflicting concerns.

Chapter 9: Facilitating critical discussion

This chapter examines the ways in which reflective journal writing can be used to promote critical discussion in small group tutorials. It was found that reflective writing served as a valuable stimulus for discussion and that the two activities in combination led to fresh insights for students and promoted critical reflection. There is an examination of the impact upon critical discussion of variables such as disclosure ground-rules, group size, physical arrangement of classrooms, inter-group interaction and the role of the tutor. In formulating arrangements for journal writing and tutorials, it was often found to be necessary to develop an intelligent working position between extreme arrangements which were apparently dichotomous.

Part IV: The nature of reflection

This part returns to the discussion of the nature of reflection which began with the literature review in Chapter 1. The examination of the theory on reflection is complemented by the results of a naturalistic study of the data gathered from reflective journals, student interviews and other material.

Chapter 10: The affective dimension of reflection

The work reported in this chapter examined the affective comments students made about the process of reflection. In initial attempts to engage in reflective thinking, it was common for students to express discomfort. The teaching and learning process was foreign to them, as the teaching was less directive than the approach they were used to. Some also had a conception of knowledge which hindered the development of reflective judgement. The process of changing perspective was often quite disturbing for the students but it could be aided by support from a group of student peers or facilitative tutors. Once students felt more confident about reflecting upon practice, their affective statements usually became more positive. There was appreciation of both success in engaging in reflective thinking and the value brought to their practice by reflection upon it.

Chapter 11: Triggers for reflection

This chapter examines triggers for reflection. A hierarchical classification scheme was used to classify information on triggers to reflection in a qualitative database. The classification scheme is used to illustrate a number of issues which emerged from the analysis.

- Reflection can occur through stimuli other than problems or disturbances to the normal routine.
- The stimuli may be encouraged or arranged.
- Reflection can be both an individual and a group activity.
- Group discussion can serve well as a spur to reflection.
- Reflection can and does take place in an academic environment. This includes the theory part of programmes and not just the professional practice component. Research for this book revealed several strategies, such as questioning, discussing and journal writing, for promoting fruitful reflection.
- Reflection is a broader concept than that portrayed in some literature on the topic which tends to take a compartmentalised view referring only to the context of professional practice.

Chapter 12: Reflections on reflection

This chapter draws together threads throughout the book which explore and investigate the construct of reflection. It presents conclusions on the nature of reflection and also draws together overall conclusions about the role and nature of reflective teaching and learning in professional education.

Part I
Introduction

Chapter 1
The nature of reflection

David Kember, Frances Kam Yuet Wong and Ella Yeung

Introduction

To introduce the concept of reflection we will draw upon an activity which we have used for this purpose in workshops on reflection. Those attending the workshop were asked to think about what they had done in their professional work the previous day and to consider:

- the tasks they performed
- the cases they dealt with and
- the judgements they made

The terminology used here is appropriate for a workshop for healthcare professionals but it would not be difficult to substitute suitable phrasing for architects, lawyers, teachers, or those from any other profession.

Having listed their activities, participants were asked to decide how they knew what to do or the basis for their actions. They were asked to allocate each activity to one of three categories:

- they followed procedures taught in their training/degree course
- they made some use of knowledge learnt during their course
- their action was not based upon knowledge specifically acquired during their training

The reader might try this activity before reading further and even if nothing is written down, at least try to think of some of the activities of yesterday and attempt to determine the basis for the action taken. This will almost certainly give a similar result to that obtained by those attending the workshops. Surprisingly few of the actions of professionals are normally allocated to the first category, i.e. of following procedures taught in their training. Most of those who attempt this activity attribute a reasonable proportion of their activities to the second category – professionals do seem to make some use of the knowledge base gained during their education. However, workshop participants always have some, and often a sizeable proportion, of their activities assigned to the final category, i.e. their action was not based upon knowledge specifically acquired during their training.

What does this mean? Are these professional courses teaching the wrong things? It is possible that there has been a predominant approach to professional education which has not equipped graduates well for practising their trade. It seems most unlikely that this is the main reason since the participants in the workshops have come from a variety of professions and have obtained their professional education from numerous universities and colleges in several countries. It seems more likely that the responses to this workshop activity reveal something about the nature of professional practice.

'Messy' problems

The nature of cases and problems tackled by professionals has been variously described as messy, wicked, ill-defined, indeterminate or 'occupying the swampy lowland' (Schön, 1983). This means that first, the problems themselves need to be identified. They can be defined in more than one way: one professional may examine a case or situation and define the problem in a particular way, whereas another could see quite different problems needing to be tackled. Issues need to be addressed with a view to problem framing or problem posing rather than problem solving.

An example of a messy problem from the field of occupational therapy is the arrangement of desks in a primary school classroom for children in wheelchairs. Issues that have to be considered include space planning, teaching style, cost implications, parental demand, and the requirements of the disability discrimination ordinance.

One approach to providing access is to redesign classrooms for more open space and fewer desks or tables. This might have implications for the designer and architect in terms of layout of rooms, for the administration in terms of admissions, and for the teacher in terms of style of teaching, since there may be legal implications if the school does not comply with legislation.

In designing the school the architect must take into account financial implications, e.g. the cost of lifts to upper floors; the environmental implications, e.g. change from traditional desks; and other diverse concerns of parents and teachers. An occupational therapist should be consulted on access issues.

An open plan classroom accessible for all children may suggest changes to areas for stimulation, the book corner, floor play space, height of desks, computer stands and counters, access to storage, and space for specialist teaching. Other innovative classroom layouts may be considered.

Even if some measure of agreement can be reached over the nature of the problem and the aspects involved, there will not be an ideal solution. There will often be conflicting tensions – a solution may have positive consequences for one aspect of the problem but negative repercussions on others.

A perfect classroom design which is ideal for all students may cost so much that approval from the governors will not be forthcoming.

Nursing example

A further example showing the ill-defined nature of the issues in professional practice is taken from nursing. It demonstrates a multi-faceted problem with no ideal solution. In the clinical setting, a nurse may encounter a situation where the son of a critically ill woman is shouting at the nurses, accusing the health care team of not trying their best to save his mother's life. The nurse may deal with this situation in a variety of ways, largely dependent on how he or she interprets the situation.

One solution to the problem is to remove the son from the ward immediately because he is disturbing other patients. Another possibility is to ignore the son because the nurse thinks he is making unreasonable accusations about the healthcare team. However, the nurse may see that patients are entitled to assert their rights and so may direct the son to the Patient Relations Department to file a complaint. On the other hand, the nurse might view the reaction of the son as a sign of him not accepting the prognosis of his mother. This interpretation would then result in the nurse trying to explain the situation to the son.

These four possible actions that can be taken by the nurse demonstrate that in a single incident multi-faceted issues can emerge. Many variables must be taken into account since the aspects of an issue are likely to involve several viewpoints.

The event can be interpreted as a ward management problem, in which case keeping the ward in order and peaceful is most important. Or, it can be treated as a bureaucratic problem, where the son is referred to different departments for further help. The nurse must understand affective behaviour and psychology and use therapeutic communication skills to deal with the problem.

There is clearly no one ideal solution to this situation. The best starting point is perhaps to frame the problem, rather than a solution since after all, a good solution comes from asking a good question. The use of bureaucratic measures in referring the son to seek help from other personnel or departments in the hospital may not help to alleviate the son's anger immediately. In fact his frustration might even escalate. However, this referral may be needed at some point when dealing with the son's anger. Perhaps the implementation of effective communication by the nurse is sufficient to solve the problem. The welfare of a single patient needs to be considered but so too does that of the other patients. In such cases, keeping the ward peaceful and orderly is necessary.

Technical rationality

In his influential book, *The Reflective Practitioner*, Donald Schön (1983) described the nature of professional practice and in *Educating the Reflective Practitioner* (1987) he argued that reflection is not well understood by those educating future professionals. He believed that the predominant technical-rational approach to professional education did not take into account that professional practice must deal with messy problems.

Schön argued that the predominant paradigm in professional schools in universities was the logical positivist one of the pure sciences. Students are taught a body of knowledge with much coming from the pure or traditional disciplines, considered to be building blocks for applied science or the more professionally oriented courses. In these, practice was often taught as clearly defined procedures with problems and assignments usually being artificial academic examples which were well defined and had identifiable correct answers.

It is probable that many of the participants in the workshop sessions had also been taught in courses which assumed a technical-rational approach. This would partly explain why participants felt that much of their practice was not based upon what they had learnt in their professional education. Whatever the nature of their professional education, though, any professional would find that it did not cover many of the tasks they attempt because of the messy nature of professional practice. In *Educating the Reflective Practitioner,* Schön (1987) argued for alternative approaches to professional education based upon a more realistic image of the work of professionals.

Reflection – the alternative to technical rationality

Schön (1983) believed that much of the routine work of professionals is tacit. Situations are dealt with and judgements made, without the professional thinking deeply about the criteria underlying the decision reached or the procedures followed. In standard cases, professionals display an almost unconscious routine which Schön calls *knowing-in-action.*

Because *knowing-in-action* is employed, many professionals or experts at it find it so difficult to articulate the processes they use in their practice. It is not unusual to hear practitioners say: 'I can do it easily myself but I find it hard to explain to you how I do it'; or 'I'm sure this is the right way to do it but I'm not sure why that is.'

Schön (1983, p. 50) clearly recognises, however, that all professional practice is not governed by knowing-in-action, acknowledging that there is an engagement with reflection stating that:

'... both ordinary people and professional practitioners often think about what they are doing, sometimes even while doing it. They may ask themselves, for example, "What features do I notice when I recognise this thing? What are the criteria by which I make this judgement? What procedures am I enacting when I perform this skill? How am I framing the problem that I am trying to solve?" Usually reflection on knowing-in-action goes together with reflection on the stuff at hand. There is some puzzling, or troubling, or interesting phenomenon with which the individual is trying to deal. As he tries to make sense of it, he also reflects on the understandings which he surfaces, criticises, restructures and embodies in further action.'

Schön (1983, p. 61) called this second type of thinking *reflection-in-action*, with the more experienced professional also reflecting upon the more routine aspects of practice. The act is essentially one of reflecting upon past activities.

'Practitioners do reflect *on* their knowing-in-practice. Sometimes in the relative tranquillity of a post-mortem, they think back on a project they have undertaken, a situation they have lived through, and they explore the understandings they have brought to the handling of the case. They may do this in a mood of idle speculation, or in a deliberate effort to prepare themselves for future cases.'

It is this ability to reflect on practice which students should develop in professional courses. The main theme of this book hinges on what the authors have learned about how to teach and design courses so that students become adept at reflecting upon their practice.

What is reflection?

What is perhaps surprising, in spite of the wide interest in reflection and the volumes written about it, is that the concept is ill-defined. Formal definitions are not easy to find as has been observed by Atkins & Murphy (1993) and Sparks-Langer, Simmons & Pasch (1990) among others. Many write about reflection with the apparent assumption that everyone knows what it is. However, the disparities in terminology, frames of reference, applications and usage make it clear that this assumption is not helpful.

An element of confusion surrounds the literature because the concept has become so widely and diversely used that it is now found within quite disparate contexts and based upon divergent frames of reference. Within one context there may be a number of writers who establish a set of terminology, unaware that those who operate within a different context are using similar terminology but with different meanings. The concept of reflection has also been approached from quite different knowledge bases. These bases range from casual observation or everyday experience to the rather daunting theoretical treatises of Habermas. Not surprisingly, these extreme starting points lead to a divergence both of views of the constructs and outcomes.

This point can be substantiated by recalling the assignment of taking from our library the number of books referred to in this chapter. This meant going to three floors of the library and visiting several sections, which were well separated by both physical distance and entries in the catalogue. The point is not the legwork involved in examining the literature for a book, but the diversity of fields which have contributed to the understanding of the concept of reflection. The books all had perfectly logical classifications but were spread around various sections of the library (see Table 1.1).

Table 1.1   A framework for reviewing the literature

Context	Orientation	Outcomes	Principal writers
General	Initial development of the concept of reflection	Description of reflective thinking	Dewey
College learning	Reflection as dealing with ill-defined problems	Description and classification of developmental stages	King & Kitchener Perry
Professional practice and education	Understanding professional practice	Description of the decision-making process by professionals	Schön
Adult education	Theoretical development	Classification of types of reflection	Mezirow van-Manen
Adult and student-centred learning	Experiential	Models of reflective thinking	Boud, Keogh & Walker Jarvis
Health science education	Developing reflective practitioners	Richer descriptions of reflection in context	Johns Atkins & Murphy

Because of the number of citations and their disparate nature, it is not possible to perform a comprehensive review of the literature since such a review would be a mammoth task and a rapidly growing one. What is more significant is whether much would be gained by such a review. Without a clear definition as a starting point and any measure of agreement on the nature of reflection, a comprehensive review would result simply in confusion and contradiction.

Instead, we will discuss the work of a limited number of writers whose research is highly regarded and has been cited and utilised by others. In order to make some sense of the alternative contexts we have attempted to indicate the background of the work. As will become apparent, most of the selected material forms the foundation for work in subsequent chapters.

When studying the literature on reflection, five main threads were identified which will be considered in some detail in this chapter.

- A definition of reflection and a more detailed description of its nature is a necessary starting point.
- As the treatment of reflection has become bound up with its context, it seems necessary to refer to this and to deal particularly with reflection in our two principal contexts of academia and professional practice.
- Our book is directed towards the health professions so there is a need to look at the more pertinent work in this area.
- As various writers have distinguished levels, types or categories of reflection, there needs to be a discussion of these.
- There have also been several attempts to discuss the mechanism by which people reflect or to develop models of the processes involved in reflective thinking.

These points are discussed at pertinent stages throughout the book. Some are covered within one of the contextual areas listed in Table 1.1, others relate to several areas.

Definitions of reflection

John Dewey (1859–1952) was an influential writer of educational thought and practice who stressed its social importance and advocated student-centred learning. He is considered to have initiated the concept of reflective thinking as an aspect of learning and education, defining it as:

> 'active, persistent and careful consideration of any belief or supposed form of knowledge in the light of the grounds that support it and the further conclusion to which it tends.'
> (Dewey, 1933, p. 9)

He saw two aspects to the process of reflective thinking:

> 'Reflective thinking, in distinction from other operations to which we apply the name of thought, involves (1) a state of doubt, hesitation, perplexity, mental difficulty, in which thinking originates, and (2) an act of searching, hunting, inquiring, to find material that will resolve the doubt, settle and dispose of the perplexity.'
> (Dewey, 1933, p.12).

He also introduced a distinction, which has endured, between *critical reflection* and less considered reflection. He argued that a person who was not sufficiently critical might reach a hasty conclusion without examining all the possible outcomes.

Dewey also argued that the development of reflective thinking should be an educational aim. His philosophical work is persuasively argued and indeed his position may be even more pertinent today than it was when written. The pace of technological change and the volume of available current information places an even greater premium upon the need to develop the ability of critical reflective thinking.

Two further definitions of reflection consistent with Dewey's are given by Boud, Keogh & Walker (1985) and Boyd & Fales (1983).

'Reflection in the context of learning is a generic term for those intellectual and affective activities in which individuals engage to explore their experiences in order to lead to new understandings and appreciation.'

(Boud, Keogh & Walker, 1985, p. 19)

'Reflective learning is the process of internally examining and exploring an issue of concern, triggered by an experience, which creates and clarifies meaning in terms of self, and which results in a changed conceptual perspective.'

(Boyd & Fales, 1983, p. 100)

These two definitions are moving towards the context of professional practice in that both view experience as the touchstone for reflection. In Dewey's original work, reflective thinking is placed in a wide context, however there has been a recent tendency by many to reserve it for the context of professional practice.

Reflective judgement

The work of Patricia King and Karen Kitchener is sited in the context of college education where they spent many years investigating students' beliefs about knowledge. They acknowledge that their work on reflective judgement (1994) follows Dewey's (1933) writing on reflective thinking. King & Kitchener see reflective judgement as the ability to deal with ill-structured problems. Such problems were discussed at the beginning of this chapter with the conclusion that the work of professionals involves dealing with messy problems. However, King & Kitchener operate within the different context of college education. Their work demonstrated that students' ability to cope with college depends upon the development of sufficiently sophisticated beliefs about knowledge and a recognition that issues can be ill-defined and demand reflective judgements.

King & Kitchener's model of reflective judgement takes into account cognitive development and contends that the ability to recognise and deal with ill-defined problems depends on beliefs about knowledge. This model has seven stages characterised by increasingly sophisticated assumptions about knowledge which are accompanied by a developing ability to reflect upon ill-structured problems.

The initial three stages are pre-reflective. Stages four and five are quasi-reflective, while in stages six and seven reflective thinking is achieved and the existence of ill-structured problems is recognised. The view of knowledge for the seven stages is summarised below.

Pre-reflective

(1)   Knowledge is absolute.
(2)   Knowledge is absolute but not always immediately available. It can be obtained from authority figures or directly observed.
(3)   Knowledge is absolute in most cases but temporarily uncertain in others.

Quasi-reflective

(4)   Knowledge is uncertain as there is always an element of ambiguity in evidence.
(5)   Knowledge is personal since individuals have to interpret the evidence.

Reflective

(6)   Knowledge about ill-structured problems is constructed by evaluating evidence and the opinions of others.
(7)   Knowledge of ill-structured problems is constructed from inquiry which leads to reasonable solutions based upon evidence currently available.

King & Kitchener's work has considerable implications for courses aiming to promote reflective thinking. Sending students on a practice session and expecting them to reflect upon their practice will clearly be frustrating for all concerned if students are in one of the pre-reflective stages. Even for those in the quasi-reflective stages the venture may not be particularly fruitful.

Results from King & Kitchener are given on a scale of 1 to 7 corresponding to the seven levels above. In their analysis of levels of reflective judgement, King and Kitchener report mean scores of around 3.5 out of 7 for college first-year students; and 4.0 out of 7 for senior students (King & Kitchener, 1994a, pp. 224–5), implying that the average senior is still at a quasi-reflective stage of development and as these are mean scores there must be many at pre-reflective stages.

Students generally develop through the reflective stages during the college years, though perhaps not as much as one might expect. The title of King & Kitchener's (1994) book, though, is *Developing Reflective Judgement* suggesting that there is a role for faculty in assisting students to make the transition through the developmental stages until they are capable of reflective judgement. It is one of the major contentions of this book that it is necessary for teachers to pay attention to the development of curricula in the theoretical elements of courses so that students are equipped to reflect upon their practice in the practice element.

The reflective judgement model is one of a number of developmental models of intellectual capacity. The one which has probably been most widely cited in application to university students is that of Perry (1970; 1988). Perry characterised students' cognitive and intellectual development by nine observed positions ranging from the unswerving belief in the correctness of authorities, through a more relativistic understanding, to the ability to evolve and evaluate personal commitments. Perry (1988) also saw a role for the teacher to assist students to develop through these positions by combining challenges with support.

Deep and surface learning

Students' approaches to learning are another set of constructs derived from research in higher education. Students were categorised as employing either a deep or a surface approach (Marton & Säljö, 1976). When using a deep approach, the intention was to seek the underlying meaning of a text. By contrast, the use of a surface approach saw students concentrating upon the text itself.

Approaches to learning and reflection are not commonly considered in the same work, but there is an indirect relationship. Students who employ a surface approach cannot be thinking reflectively. Thinking reflectively must imply a deep approach but it is possible to utilise a deep approach to learning without necessarily reflecting upon practice, as the topic could be a theoretical one, divorced from the experience of the student.

It has been shown (see Ramsden, 1992, and Biggs, 1999 for general treatments) that a range of factors within the broad teaching environment can influence which approach a student employs for a particular learning task. Students can be induced to employ a surface approach by factors such as the following:

- assessment which demands purely recall
- excessive workload
- over-formal relationships with teaching staff
- didactic teaching methods which provide little opportunity for interaction or activity
- teaching which fails to capture the interest of students

Metacognition

Another higher order thinking process which might be compared to reflection is metacognition. The term has been used to refer to two somewhat separate phenomena: knowledge about cognition; and regulation of cognition (Baker & Brown, 1984). The first is concerned with a person's knowledge about his or her own cognitive resources. If the learner is aware of what is needed to perform effectively, then it is possible for him or her to take steps to meet the demands of a learning situation more adequately. If, however, the learner is not aware of his or her limitations or the complexity of the task at hand, then the learner can hardly be expected to deal properly with the type of typically ill-defined issues with which professionals deal.

The second phenomenon of the regulation of cognition is used by a learner when attempting to solve a problem. The indices of metacognition include checking the outcome of an attempt to solve a problem, planning one's next move, monitoring the effectiveness of any attempted action, and testing, revising and evaluating one's strategies for learning. Furthermore Baker & Brown (1984) state that effective learning requires an active monitoring of one's own cognitive activities.

Metacognition is clearly a reflective process. The act of monitoring one's own cognition requires self-reflection. Again, though, the two constructs are not the same. It is important, however, to be aware of the literature relating to both approaches to learning and metacognition when looking at the meaning of reflection.

Reflective practice

The literature concerned with the reflective practice component, and in particular the influential work of Schön (1983; 1987) has been referred to earlier in this chapter. It is, though, instructive to examine the relationship between the literature on educating the reflective practitioner with that reviewed above on developing reflective judgement.

Surprisingly there seems to be little relationship at all. King & Kitchener (1994) do not reference Schön or many other writers from the discipline of either adult education or the health sciences, whose work is dealt with in the remainder of this chapter. Apart from common acknowledgements to the pioneering work of Dewey, there is little overlap between the references in the texts by Schön and King & Kitchener. Despite each of them having extensive bibliographies, there is little in common between them, possibly because they originate from different disciplinary backgrounds.

It is interesting that the work of King & Kitchener (1994) relating to reflective judgement does not find application in the field of professional education and the work related to educating professionals makes little reference to the literature concerned with developing reflective judgement in general education. This is probably because the major references in the literature to reflective practice refer to the practice setting.

Compartmentalising literature reviews by discipline area seems to be quite common. The work on reflection in the adult education area draws mainly upon the work of other adult educators. Similarly most of those in the health sciences show a preference for work from those in their own discipline area. The outcome of such compartmentalising is limiting as insights from those in other disciplines would often be relevant, particularly if adaptations were to be made.

Limitations of Schön's work

Schön's work has been criticised for its limitations. The two major areas which have been highlighted are the narrow view of reflection and the lack of variety in the types of teaching situations described.

Greenwood (1998) is one who has criticised the limitations of Schön's model by pointing out that it only involves two components of reflective practice, that is, reflection-in-action and reflection-on-action. Greenwood noted particularly the failure to recognise the importance of reflection-before-action. Reflection-before-action involves thinking through what one intends to do before doing it. This reduces the chances of making errors. Greenwood's view of reflection is more in line with Boud, Keogh & Walker's model (1985) which emphasises preparation for experience as well as the re-evaluation of the experience.

Eraut (1995) questioned the construct of reflection-in-action by pointing out that he had observed little evidence of reflection-in-action in the complex interplay of a typical classroom setting. This observation is interesting as in most courses which claim to promote reflective practice, the stress is upon reflection-on-action.

Schön's work on educating reflective practitioners (1983) is limited, in that examples of educating potential professionals are in the context of a professional practice situation such as a studio. The prominent example is an architectural studio where a student learns to design under the guidance of a coach. Other examples are of the teaching of psycho-analytic practice to a resident by a supervisor, and a musical performance master class in which a master teacher guides an advanced student. The limitation will be all too obvious to most readers who do not have the luxury of being able to hold extensive individual counselling sessions. As Schön's examples deal with a form of education which is impractical for current higher education practice, the development of guidelines for teaching and developing curricula for reflective practice has been effectively left to others. This book, is therefore, a major contribution to filling this breach.

A further limitation of Schön's contribution to education is that all his examples refer to the practice situation in a studio and make no reference to the theoretical element of the large majority of professional programmes. Similarly, most of the literature on reflective practice deals with the period of professional experience which students undertake. Very little covers the other non-practice parts of courses which are normally considered to be the theory element.

This divide is interesting in that one of the most widely cited rationales for reflective practice in professional education has been concerned with bridging the theory/practice gap (e.g. Clarke, 1986; Tichen & Binnie, 1992; Conway, 1994). It is one of the major contentions of this book that the gulf will not be bridged if reflection-on-practice is confined to the professional practice component.

The work of King & Kitchener (1994) also raises the question of whether students are prepared and able to engage in reflection upon their practice. They will not be able to achieve this unless they have reached the appropriate developmental stage of reflective judgement. There is little to be gained from sending students to reflect upon the ill-defined issues of professional practice if they still view knowledge in cut and dried terms, as they will not be able even to recognise that practice consists of messy problems. The development of students towards appropriate conceptions of knowledge and to higher stages in reflective judgement is surely a concern of the theory element of courses.

Of importance to the academic community, is the recognition that reflection can take place in an academic context and not just in an environment of professional practice. For programmes of professional practice, reflection can take place in both the university and the professional practice settings. Indeed, if reflection is seen as a bridge between theory and practice, it is important that it is actively promoted within the theoretical elements of the course and not confined to the practice situation. It is also important to recognise that students frequently have unsophisticated conceptions of knowledge and are ill-equipped to engage in reflective thinking. These abilities can, though, be cultivated during academic programmes.

Types of reflection

Major contributors to widening perspectives on the nature of reflection have come from the field of adult education. Some of these have approached the work from a theoretical perspective, others have taken a more experiential view. Some of those starting from theory have derived several types or levels of reflection from their chosen framework and context. The most developed of these are perhaps those who have taken the work of Habermas (e.g. 1970; 1972; 1974) as their basic theoretical framework.

An early work which draws upon Habermas is that of van-Manen (1977). His writing related to curriculum development and discussed the effect of epistemological assumptions upon curricula. His argument was that it was only through critical reflection that important curriculum issues could be addressed.

One of the best developed expositions on the levels or types of reflection comes from the work of Jack Mezirow, who has written extensively on the subject of reflection as an essential component of his model of transformative learning for adults. The following section is principally derived from Mezirow (1991), of which Chapter 4 is most central to defining reflection. Other works by Mezirow (1977; 1985; 1992) also contributed to clarifying the meaning of important constructs as does his more recent work (Mezirow, 1998).

The influence of Habermas and critical theory is readily apparent in Mezirow's work. As such it has a political agenda because critical theory was developed alongside Marxism. In our discussion of the work we have not drawn upon this as our interest is on reflection within an educational and professional context.

Mezirow separates reflective action from non-reflective action. While being principally interested in reflective thinking, it is helpful to first distinguish what is not reflection so as to better define what is reflection. Three types of non-reflective action are distinguished: habitual action, thoughtful action and introspection.

Habitual action

Habitual action is that which has been learnt previously and, through frequent use, becomes an activity which is performed automatically or with little conscious thought. Examples are riding a bicycle or using a keyboard. Habitual actions are clearly not reflective, though much professional practice seems to become habitual for more experienced practitioners.

Thoughtful action

Thoughtful action makes use of existing knowledge, without attempting to appraise that knowledge, so learning remains within pre-existing meaning schemes and perspectives. Much of the 'book learning' which takes place in universities is best classified as thoughtful action. Students can try to reach an understanding of the concepts without relating them to their own experiences. Thoughtful action can be described as a cognitive process.

Thoughtful action differs from habitual action in that the latter does not require thinking about the action while performing it. When we ride a bike we do not normally think about the technique or mechanics of riding. For professionals in their everyday practice, much of their work can become fairly routine, in which case they tend not to reflect upon their actions. Their normal mode of operation becomes thoughtful action in Mezirow's terminology, or 'knowing-in-practice' according to Schön's work (1983, pp. 61–62).

> 'As practice becomes more repetitive and routine, and as knowing-in-practice becomes increasingly tacit and spontaneous, the practitioner may miss important opportunities to think about what he is doing. Through reflection, he can surface and criticise the tacit understandings that have grown up around the repetitive experiences of a specialised practice, and can make new sense of the situations of uncertainty or uniqueness which he may allow himself to experience. Practitioners do reflect on their knowing-in-practice.'

It is only when cases occur which do not fit within the normally experienced framework that reflection becomes necessary.

Introspection

Unlike thoughtful action, which is concerned with cognition, introspection lies in the affective domain. It refers to feelings or thoughts about ourselves. The feelings can be personal, such as recognising that we feel happy, upset or bored with something. Introspection can involve the recognition that we have feelings towards others, such as liking or disliking them. It does not, however, encompass decisions about how or why these feelings developed since that becomes reflective thinking. Introspection remains at the level of recognition or awareness of these feelings.

Mezirow (1991, p. 107) regarded introspection as not reflective because it involves no attempt to re-examine or test the validity of prior knowledge. Others, such as Boud & Walker (1993), have observed an affective dimension associated with reflection. The affective dimension of reflection and the role of introspection are explored in Chapter 10.

Reflection

When Mezirow himself considers reflection, the influence of critical theory upon his work becomes apparent. He defines reflection as:

'Reflection involves the critique of assumptions about the content or process of problem solving. . . . The critique of premises or presuppositions pertains to problem *posing* as distinct from problem *solving*. Problem posing involves making a taken-for-granted situation problematic, raising questions regarding its validity.'

(Mezirow, 1991, p. 105)

Mezirow then proceeds to subdivide reflection into three categories of content, process and premise reflection. We interpreted content and process reflection as being equivalent in level. The two are distinguishable in terms of the subject matter of the reflection. Content reflection being concerned with *what*, while process examines *how*.

Mezirow (1991, p. 107–8) defines content reflection as: 'Reflection on *what* we perceive, think, feel or act upon.' He defines process reflection as the method or manner in which we think: 'Examination of *how* one performs the functions of perceiving, thinking, feeling, or acting and an assessment of efficacy in performing them.'

Premise reflection

Premise reflection is seen as a higher level of reflection because it is through premise reflection that we can transform our meaning framework as it opens the possibility of perspective transformation. As Mezirow (1991, p. 108) defines it: 'Premise reflection involves us becoming aware of *why* we perceive, think, feel or act as we do.'

It is the premise reflection which borrows most from the foundation of Mezirow's work on critical theory (Mezirow, 1981) and the writing of Habermas (e.g. 1970; 1972; 1974). To undergo a perspective transformation, it is necessary to recognise that many of our actions are governed by a set of beliefs and values which have been almost unconsciously assimilated from a particular environment. Premise reflection then requires a critical review of presuppositions from conscious and unconscious prior learning and an understanding of their consequences.

Conventional wisdom and ingrained assumptions are hard to change, in part, because they become so deeply embedded that we become unaware that they are assumptions or even that they exist. Mezirow (1991, p. 110) clearly recognises the difficulty of perspective transformation, stating that 'It must involve a hiatus in which a problem becomes redefined so that action may be redirected.'

Premise reflection is, therefore, unlikely to occur frequently. This would be particularly true of topics which are central to our main activities as these have the most numerous and the most deep-seated beliefs. Perspective transformation is easier if the topic is more peripheral to the main interest and activity of the person.

Mezirow's recognition of perspective transformation as a more profound level of reflection has parallels in the work of others. Dewey's (1933) distinction between critical and less considered reflection was mentioned earlier. It is the term *critical reflection* which has more commonly been used to describe the deeper form of reflection.

Models of reflective thinking

Another aspect of reflection, which has achieved some attention in the literature, is the mechanism by which reflective thinking takes place. Of the various attempts to model reflective thinking, the well developed model by Boud, Keogh & Walker (1985) to be one of the most useful. This model was later refined by Boud & Walker (1991) and there are further comments on the nature of reflection in Boud & Walker (1998).

Reflection has been defined by Boud, Keogh & Walker (1985) as 'an important human activity in which people recapture their experience, think about it, mull it over and evaluate it'. The central point of reflection in learning is experience.

The reflective process involves both feelings and cognition which are closely interrelated and interactive. The feelings may be positive or negative. They cue the individual to respond at the initial stage of the reflective process. Intensive personal feelings are also present towards the end stage of the reflective process (Boud, Keogh & Walker, 1985). They further state that as an outcome of reflection, the individual is enabled to act upon his or her convictions with the commitment to action becoming the life-force of the individual. The cognitive activities include making inferences, discriminating and associating relationships, and validating assumptions.

Boud, Keogh & Walker also depict a model of the reflective process in which they suggest the key elements of the process. The model explains that as an individual encounters an experience, so he or she responds. The reflective process is initiated when the individual returns to the experience, recollecting what has taken place and replaying the experience. Then re-evaluation takes place. There are four elements in the process of re-evaluation:

(1) Association – relating new data to that which is already known.
(2) Integration – seeking relationships among the data.
(3) Validation – determining the authenticity of the ideas and feelings which have resulted.
(4) Appropriation – making knowledge one's own.

The outcomes of reflection may include development of a new perspective or changes in behaviour. The synthesis, validation and appropriation of knowledge are part of the reflective process, but they can be outcomes as well. Boud, Keogh & Walker suggest that the elements be separated just to draw attention to the various features in the process. The elements do not proceed in a linear sequence, nor are they independent of each other. Some stages can be omitted or some of the elements can at times be compressed.

Models of learning

Peter Jarvis is, like David Boud, a professor in the field of adult education. He has developed a model of learning which is perhaps broader than the previous model as it encompasses non-learning and non-reflective learning as well as reflective learning. The starting point for the model was Kolb's (1984) learning cycle. Jarvis, though, felt this was rather simplistic for a process as complex as learning so he invited seminar participants to construct models to describe their own learning experiences.

After extensive refinement through this process, the outcome was a more complex model of learning (Jarvis, 1987; 1992; 1995). The model divides learning into three categories of response to experience: non-learning, non-reflective learning and reflective learning. Each category then has three types of learning associated with it. For example, the three types of reflective learning are contemplation, reflective skills learning and experimental learning. Including nine types of learning within the same model makes it more comprehensive but at the same time more complex.

The nine elements start with the person and the situation. Each of the nine types of learning is described by a different route through some sub-set of the nine elements. It is impossible to deal with all the forms of learning within a brief review but to give one example, the path in the contemplation form of reflection takes the following steps:

- person
- situation
- experience
- reasoning and reflecting
- evaluation
- memorisation
- person changed and more experienced

The four final steps are shown as a two way process. The process can then be cyclical or iterative.

The strength of Jarvis's model is that reflection is recognised as being related to other forms of thinking and learning. It is further broadened by being widely applicable, rather than restricted to particular domains. The breadth of applicability, though, presumably involved a trade-off in that the model does not provide as rich a description of reflective thinking itself compared to some of the other models examined.

Health science education

The two highlighted limitations of Schön's work have created openings for others to pursue. Those involved in the health professions have been active both in widening the perspective on the nature of reflection and in trying to show how students might be taught to become reflective practitioners using methods which are more realistic for the cash strapped universities of today. This chapter considers two attempts to widen the characterisation of reflection.

Johns's guided framework of reflection

A recent model, developed in the nineties, has been the result of the work of Christopher Johns from the field of nurse education. Johns based the development of his work on Carper's (1978) four patterns of knowing. He believes that reflection is a deliberate and structured activity, so much so that he has developed a guided framework of reflection.

Johns asserts that the existing norms of nursing practice constrain the practitioners' caring potential, and guided reflection facilitates the challenge of these norms (Johns,

1996a). Before elaborating on Johns' guided framework of reflection, it would be helpful to briefly review the work of Carper which underpins Johns's model.

Johns (1995a; 1995b) cites the work of Barbara Carper (1978) who outlined four ways of knowing: the empirical, the personal, the ethical and the aesthetic. The *empirical* facilitates the practitioner to view the situation according to some rule or law. The situation described is stereotypical, and the outcome of the situation is predictable. The *personal* recognises the engagement of self in the practice setting. There is an understanding that working with patients is often difficult and stressful. The *ethical* is concerned with managing value conflicts when dealing with clinical situations that require value judgement. The 'aesthetic' is grasping the nature of a clinical situation where information and meaning for those involved are interpreted, the desired outcomes are envisioned and the achieved outcomes are reflected. Johns believes that this reflects the fullness of the nursing situation. He compares Carper's model with the nursing process – a common problem solving approach used by nurses, but criticised by Johns as linear and separate. Unlike the nursing process, Carper's model promotes a more dynamic inter-personal process of caring in nursing practice than nursing process (Johns, 1996a).

Why must reflection be guided? According to Johns, practitioners are socialised and accustomed to conventional ways of practice. They take for granted the everyday world and do not necessarily see the need to reflect on practice. Johns therefore alleges that practitioners need guidance to help them see beyond the reality, and envisage new ways of practice (Johns, 1995a). Reflection, it can be argued, involves the process of *unlearning*. The guided reflection helps to create space for individuals to reflect-in-action and develop expertise and confidence (Johns, 1996b). He illustrates how he guided the student through reflection by providing reflective cues based on the structured reflection model he developed. In the process, he constantly analysed the supervision dialogue within the guided reflection relationships to enable the practitioner to unfold situations that are present within everyday practice. By assimilating learning through reflection with existing personal knowledge, the practitioner can then respond to new situations within a changed perspective (Johns, 1995b). The process involves personal deconstruction and reconstruction, and learning through reflection. It is a process that encompasses enlightenment, empowerment and emancipation. Enlightenment is to understand the self in the context of practice. Empowerment is to have the courage and commitment to take necessary action. Emancipation is to liberate oneself from previous ways of being so as to achieve a more desirable way of practice. Reflection frees the practitioner's senses and makes caring visible (Johns, 1996b). Through reflection, the practitioner can appreciate self in the context of the work environment. Johns acknowledges that practitioners may feel powerless to take action to change the reality, and he asserts that practitioners need both challenge and support to confront practice as exposed through reflection on experience (Johns, 1995b).

Atkins & Murphy model

It is useful to examine another model of reflective thinking at this stage. Atkins & Murphy (1993) claim that their model results from a review and synthesis of the work of Mezirow, 1981; Schön, 1983; Boud, Keogh & Walker, 1985; and Powell, 1989 on this topic. Note that these authors span several of the frameworks identified within the literature. The review was also undertaken from the perspective of health science professionals, the discipline area on which this book is based.

Atkins & Murphy claim to have discovered in the above writers a common understanding of the reflective processes. They all identified the process of reflection as the internal examination of self, which results in a changed conceptual perspective. The authors divided the key elements of reflective process into three stages:

(1) awareness of uncomfortable feelings and thoughts
(2) critical analysis
(3) new perspective

Awareness of uncomfortable feelings and thoughts are often a trigger point when one realises that the knowledge possessed is insufficient to explain what is happening in a unique situation. This self-realisation results in a sense of inner discomfort as described by Boyd & Fales (1983). The authors identify that self-awareness and the ability to describe the salient features of the experience (verbally and/ or in writing) as the essential skills required at this stage.

Critical analysis involves an examination of the feelings and knowledge of the situation and may include aesthetic, personal, moral and empirical knowledge (Atkins &

Murphy, 1993). Such examination allows the person to analyse his/her existing knowledge and may sometimes provide an explanation of the unique situation. It is also possible that the analysis may involve the examination or generation of new knowledge. This is similar to the four critical thought processes suggested by Boud, Keogh & Walker (1985) and consists of association, integration, validation and appropriation.

As a result of an exploration of a unique situation, new perspectives of the situation may develop. The integration of new knowledge with previous knowledge, i.e. synthesis and evaluation, are crucial to the development of a new perspective. Mezirow (1981) described this stage as perspective transformation in which learning takes place.

Subsequent analysis of this model has shown it to be over simplistic. Nevertheless it is worth including at this stage as it does suggest the key elements in reflection. There seems however to be much more to reflection than just these three steps.

Summary

As with the first chapter in most books, we have taken steps to define our main topic of reflection and review the relevant literature. To impose some logical structure on the mass of material, we have ordered the work in terms of its originating context and the types of outcome towards which the authors work. The review has been limited to a few of the more prominent writers on the topic and so should be seen as providing a framework to interpret the literature.

If one accepts Dewey (1933) as providing the original formulation of the idea of reflective thinking, the concept can be considered to be holistic. The work was a philosophical examination of the nature of thinking in general. This led to a treatise urging all educational programmes to see the development of reflective thinking as an aim, and perhaps as the most important aim.

Since this landmark text, a number of research traditions have emerged which examine reflection within a specific context or choose to apply it to more particular ends. The general education tradition of Dewey has been followed by King & Kitchener (1994) who see reflective judgement as developing through a number of stages in college education.

Some adult education specialists have approached reflective thinking from a theoretical standpoint and have found the work of Habermas a useful starting point. In this chapter we looked in detail at the work of Mezirow which provided a detailed description of types of reflective thinking. Others from the field of adult education have taken a more experiential starting point. From this tradition, we highlighted the model of reflective thinking developed by Boud, Keogh & Walker. Practitioners from nursing education and the other health sciences have also contributed to widening our thinking about the process of reflection with the work of Johns being particularly illuminating.

The most prominent field drawing upon the concept of reflection is currently that of the reflective practitioner in the professional practice context. The seminal writing of Schön has ensured that numerous programmes of professional education are aiming to produce reflective practitioners.

It may help in interpreting the breadth of literature on this topic to consider the tradition from which the work is derived. This should help in dealing with the differing uses of the same or similar terminology. A wider view of the topic may also make available relevant work from other traditions.

A synthesised definition of reflection

If theory is to be integrated with practice, then professional programmes need to develop students' ability to engage in reflective thinking in the theoretical elements of the courses and not leave it to the practice component. Furthermore, unless students are at a stage of development which enables them to engage in reflective judgement, they are unlikely to reflect successfully upon their practice in the practice component of programmes.

In this latter case we need to adopt a wider definition of reflection than the various authors, reviewed above, who have written about reflection with reference to a particular academic discipline or tradition. In this book we need to operate across the two most common contexts of college courses and professional practice and draws upon several of the fields in the literature. To this end we offer the following multi-faceted definition of reflection:

- The subject matter of reflection is an ill-defined problem – the type of issues and cases dealt with in professional practice.
- The process of reflection may be triggered by an unusual case or can be deliberately stimulated.

- Reflection operates through a careful re-examination and evaluation of experience, beliefs and knowledge.
- Reflection most commonly involves looking back or reviewing past actions, though competent professionals can develop the ability to reflect while engaging in their practice.
- Reflection leads to new perspectives.
- Reflection operates at a number of levels, from the highest level of critical reflection necessitating a change to deep-seated – and often unconscious – beliefs, and leads to new belief structures.
- Reflective thinking ability is reached through a developmental process linked to developing appropriate conceptions of knowledge.

Chapter 12 will return to this definition and expand it in the light of the exploration of the topic throughout the work which led to this book.

Terminology

Terminology is also relevant. Particular authors have used different terms. Again this is influenced by the context of their work and the literature to which they refer. As far as possible in this book the terminology is consistent with this existing usage, though the overlaps suggest that consistency is difficult to achieve.

Dewey (1933) wrote mainly of *reflective thinking* as a thought process which education should strive to cultivate. King & Kitchener (1994) use *reflective judgement* as a quality which college students need to develop in order to recognise and deal with ill-defined problems. Schön uses the terms *knowing-in-action, reflection-in-action* and *reflection-on-action* to refer to types of thinking pursued by *reflective practitioners* in the pursuit of their professional practice. A higher level of reflective thinking was designated by Dewey (1933) as *critical reflection* while Mezirow (1991) used the term *premise reflection*.

This book uses each of the above terms when writing of a context and usage similar to that of the authors cited. The general term reflection has been used in a wider sense to encompass the above terms in a way which is consistent with these definitions.

Chapter 2
Action research and its application to the project

David Kember, Harrison Tse and Jan McKay

Introduction

The project which resulted in this book was not planned from the outset in its final form but evolved from a number of similar, but originally separate, initiatives. These original initiatives were programme or department specific ventures to make curricula for courses or programmes more suited to the development of reflective practitioners. Loosely at least, these initiatives all had an action research format. The reason is quite simple – of the accepted research paradigms, action research is the only one to positively embrace change.

Action research

Action research has become widely accepted in the health sciences, education, management and other fields, so many texts are available to describe it and its procedures (Stenhouse, 1975; Carr & Kemmis, 1986; Elliott, 1991; McKernan, 1991; McNiff, 1992; Kember, 2000). As it was fundamental to the project on which this book is based, a brief introduction is given to its main characteristics.

There are several schools or variants of action research. These range from quite pragmatic procedures for dealing with ill-defined problems to approaches derived from critical theory, with associated political overtones as critical theory is related to Marxist calls for emancipation. There are, though, characteristics common to action research which collectively distinguish it from research conducted under positivist or interpretative paradigms. A definition of the essential components of action research by Carr & Kemmis (1986, pp. 165–166) would be widely accepted.

'It can be argued that three conditions are individually necessary and jointly sufficient for action research to be said to exist: firstly, a project takes as its subject-matter a social practice, regarding it as a form of strategic action susceptible of improvement; secondly, the project proceeds through a spiral of cycles of planning, acting, observing and reflecting, with each of these activities being systematically and self-critically implemented and interrelated; thirdly, the project involves those responsible for the practice in each of the moments of the activity, widening participation in the project gradually to include others affected by the practice, and maintaining collaborative control of the process.'

To expand further upon the nature of action research, the following features have been distilled from a number of accounts representing the major typologies (Stenhouse, 1975; Carr & Kemmis, 1986; Elliott, 1991; McKernan, 1991; McNiff, 1992). In the following section of this chapter each of these aspects of action research will be briefly discussed. Action research:

- aims towards improvement
- is a cyclical process
- incorporates reflection upon action
- involves systematic inquiry
- is concerned with social practice
- is usually a participative venture
- demands that the participants decide the topic

Perhaps the clearest distinction between action research and other modes lies in the attitude to changes to what is being researched. Other paradigms carefully avoid contaminating or perturbing the subject of their research. Action researchers set out with the avowed intention of making changes and improving their practice. Lewin (1952) and Rapoport (1970) both maintain that research should go beyond the production of books and papers to achieving social change. As such, action research has been widely applied in situations in which participants wish to improve their own practice, in fields such as education, management, social work, etc. In education it has been reasonably prevalent in the school sector but less widespread in higher education.

Action research is portrayed as a cyclical or spiral process involving steps of planning, acting, observing and reflecting, though, in practice, the steps are less discrete than they appear in pictorial representations. It is normal for a project to go through two or more cycles in an iterative process. There is provision for refinement of an initiative through a series of cycles, each incorporating lessons from previous cycles.

Inherent within the action research cycle is a need for the researchers to reflect upon their actions and their practices. The reflection is on the observations and outcomes arising from the project and on the underlying practices and beliefs of the participants. It is through this collective reflection that changes in perspective can occur. Use of a research approach with an integral reflective component is obviously highly appropriate for this particular project.

Action research is not a 'soft' or imprecise mode of research since rigorous systematic inquiry is as integral as for other paradigms. The action research cycle incorporates systematic observation and evaluation. Outcomes of systematic inquiry are made public and subjected to normal criteria for scrutiny and acceptance. Action research does, then, contribute to both social practice and the development of theory.

The title 'participative action research' has been used by some, indicating firstly that it is normally a group activity involving those affected by the topic being investigated. There may well be an attempt to widen the circle to include others involved in the practice. Some would consider it essential that action research be conducted by a group. Others, however, accept that it can be an individual reflecting on his or her practice or an individual problem-solving activity.

The term 'participative' is also indicative of the importance placed in the participation of practitioners themselves. A distinction has been made with other paradigms where it is more common for expert researchers to conduct inquiries and hand down their findings and recommendations to those in the field.

The roles of the practitioner and expert researcher also influence the subject matter of action research. It has been claimed (Stenhouse, 1975; Carr & Kemmis, 1986; Elliott, 1991; McKernan, 1991; McNiff, 1992) that educational researchers following other paradigms commonly concentrate upon theoretical issues which are of little interest or relevance to teachers. In action research, though, it is the participants or teachers who decide the subject or topic for research. It can be something they feel is interesting or important or it can be a problem they want to solve. The advocates of action research claim, therefore, that it brings theory closer to practice.

Recently, action research has emerged as an approach to enhancing the quality of teaching and learning in universities. It is one of the few strategies for quality improvement or educational development underpinned by both a theoretical framework and by practical experience (Kember & Gow, 1992; Zuber-Skerrit, 1992; Kember & Kelly, 1993; Kember & McKay, 1996).

For a more detailed account of how to apply educational action research as an approach to enhancing teaching and learning, see Kember (2000) which provides a detailed account of the nature of action research and action learning. It is a practical guide on how to conduct action research projects which aim to introduce innovation in teaching and improve the quality of student learning. Methods for evaluating projects and learning outcomes are described.

A project with five sub-projects

The project was unusual in that it developed by merging together five sub-projects. These sub-projects remained as individual entities throughout the life of the overall project, yet, at the same time they became fused together into a single broader and, in some ways deeper, project. This section describes the formulation and implemention of an action research study with a hierarchical structure of an overall project with sub-projects.

The initiative started with three originally quite independent projects in the same university faculty. Each was an action research project related to some aspect of reflective teaching for a particular course. Joint meetings were arranged for the three groups. These turned out to be valuable experiences as the participants learnt from each other's experiences. In time, the projects merged into an overall project and embraced two new initiatives. The combined project also took on other research aims described previously.

The individual issues were tackled through an action research approach. Cycles of planning, action, observation and reflection were used to test and refine components of five courses designed to promote reflection and reflective writing. Each course was the subject of an individual action research study looking at the teaching within the course and whether it facilitated student reflection. Here, we make a distinction between courses and programmes. A course refers to a discrete subject offered in specific programmes. Each course usually extends for a semester. Programmes, on the other hand, consist of a number of courses or subjects, offered over a given period of time and lead to a tertiary qualification – degree or diploma.

As five courses were examined simultaneously, comparison was possible and lessons learnt from one could be applied in others. Essentially the research consisted of five action research spirals, one for each course. As the studies proceeded simultaneously and mutual reflection developed, the spirals became intertwined. On top of this tangled web of spirals was a sixth spiral which was the cyclical processes of this overall project synthesised from the five course-based projects. This can be viewed as a spiral synthesised from and feeding back into the five course-based spirals.

The research team themselves engaged in reflection upon the outcomes of the work, the whole of the team meeting fortnightly. This facilitated comparison between courses and served as a means of passing conclusions for practice from one course to another. The critical discourse of these meetings was both an element of the project methodology and a contribution to the data. Meetings were tape-recorded and transcripts produced of useful sections of the dialogue.

The process of writing also contributed to the group's exploration of the topics. Taking Chapter 8 on reflective writing as an example, the factors which seemed to influence reflective writing were noted from the group's reflective discussions of their courses. A structure for the chapter was then prepared with headings for each of the teaching aspects which appeared to influence the degree of reflection. Those teaching each course then agreed to write notes about their course under each of the headings. These notes were collected together within the framework of the chapter as a 'patchwork quilt'.

The initial patchwork quilt served as a stimulus for considerable discussion. The notes about one course often stimulated those teaching other courses to reconsider aspects of their course which they had not included in their own notes. The attempt to synthesise conclusions from the patchwork was through collaborative critical reflection. The chapter eventually went through numerous iterative drafts, each of which provided further stimulus for collective reflection.

Data collection and analysis

During the course of the projects considerable amounts of data were gathered for the observation or evaluation facet of the action research cycle. Some class discussion sessions were tape-recorded. Interviews were held to gather information about the effectiveness of the measures for promoting reflective behaviour, the difficulties students faced in engaging in reflective writing and any benefits the students accrued from engaging in reflection-on-action in their professional practice. Data were also gathered from student journals and reports.

In Chapters 3 to 9 the data are used in conjunction with our critical reflection to derive and verify insights and conclusions about the teaching initiatives and their impact upon student learning. Typical quotations from interviews and journals are used to substantiate and illuminate some of the conclusions drawn within individual courses and from the comparison of courses.

The project used the computer programme NUD•IST (Richards & Richards, 1991) to handle the large amount of qualitative data which were gathered. The programme has facilities for indexing, text-searching, using Boolean operations on defined index nodes and combining data from several initially independent studies. It is, therefore, very effective for a project which has multiple data sources and several aims, as it facilitates searches and comparison of data.

Some of the gathered data were also used for a more detailed examination of the nature of reflection. This work took a naturalistic approach as it aimed to examine reflection from the perspective of the reflectors, in most instances the students enrolled in the courses. Essentially it looked at students' descriptions of reflection and the reflective thinking process with the aim of reaching a better understanding of the nature of reflection. The outcomes of this part of the project are described in Chapters 10 and 11.

Schön's (1983) discussion of the nature of reflection is based upon observation of, and discussion with, professionals and experienced practitioners going about their practice. This is not an easy task as much of the routine work of professionals is tacit. Cases are dealt with and judgements are made without the professional thinking deeply about the criteria underlying the decision reached or the procedures followed. In standard cases professionals display an almost unconscious routine which Schön calls *knowing-in-action*. Even when conscious reflection does take place, most professionals find it difficult to fully articulate the rationale underlying their judgement or the processes they used to arrive at a decision.

In spite of the difficulty of obtaining data directly from those engaged in reflective thinking, it is surely important to pursue this avenue. It is only through the voice of the reflector that one can reach a genuine picture of the nature and mechanism of reflection. Studies based upon the perspective of the researcher, or the theories of another, always run the danger of imposing a framework which is not inherent in the subject.

For these reasons, the study described in this chapter attempted to clarify aspects of reflective thinking through a naturalistic inquiry. The key characteristics of the naturalistic approach (Owens, 1982), as they relate to this study, are the absence of testable hypotheses and limited use of a priori theory. Rather, the theory is allowed to emerge from the data using what Glaser & Strauss (1967) refer to as 'grounded theory'. Naturalistic inquiry recognises the importance of context and sees phenomena in terms of multiple interacting relationships between the facets of the whole.

This study also recognised the importance of seeking a second order perspective (Marton, 1981; 1986). Essentially it was trying to understand the phenomenon from the perspective of the subject rather than that of the researcher. The voice of the reflector, therefore, constituted the data for the study and also formed its analytic framework. Data gathering processes were open-ended and semi-structured so as to avoid, as far as possible, imposing the framework and theories of the researchers on the reflectors.

The study used the evaluation data, gathered from the five courses, for the wider project. For this particular part of the project the NUD•IST database was searched for any statements pertaining to reflection. The research team examined the statements about reflection and eventually sorted them into a number of inter-related categories. The analysis process was initially conducted individually. Outcomes were brought back for comparison and group discussion, through which consensus was reached on the constructs and categories of significance and the next stage in refining the analysis.

The researchers started the analysis procedures by reading the written and verbal descriptions of students' reflective learning experiences so that a general understanding of their meaning could be obtained. The significant statements or textual units regarding the affective responses were extracted from the data. Individual researchers then continued to formulate the meanings from the statements and establish the formulated meanings into a set of main themes.

The researchers met and discussed the preliminary conclusions after they had completed the formulation of theme clusters. Whenever there was inconsistency among the clustering, each researcher's opinion was brought to discussion with reference to students' original narratives. At this stage, some of the theme clusters were collapsed and re-devised.

Ethical issues

There were a number of ethical issues which the projects had to address. The first was that of introducing innovations into a teaching programme. For one project the introduction of learning contracts was a voluntary affair. Both students and clinical educators were perfectly free to choose whether or not to participate in the venture. The voluntary nature of the innovation was largely adopted because of the difficulties of introducing learning contracts within each of the centres where students were allocated for clinical placements.

All other initiatives were introduced across a course for all enrolled students. The innovation was treated in the same way as any other course or curriculum development. Where necessary, approval was obtained from the relevant course committee for the original teaching plan or any subsequent modifications to it. We see the efforts to improve teaching and learning within the programmes, as ethical as any other curriculum development process, and in fact see it as unethical not to try to enhance the quality of learning and teaching.

Introducing innovations across a course, following institutional course planning procedures, is consistent with an action research approach. It also avoids the ethical and practical issues which arise if an innovation is trialled with part of a student cohort on either a voluntary basis or following some sampling design. The main ethical issue here is whether experiment or control groups are disadvantaged by receiving differing forms of instruction. There are also numerous practical problems, such as ensuring comparability, separating the groups, controlling contextual variables and keeping non-experimental conditions constant between groups (Kember, Charlesworth, Davies, McKay & Stott, 1997).

Collection of data for evaluation purposes, though, was on

a voluntary basis. In all cases the students were informed that the teaching team was trying out a new curriculum endeavour, which aimed to promote reflective learning. It was explained that alongside the curriculum innovation, the teaching team would undertake research to monitor and evaluate the effects of the new approach. The students were then asked whether their journals could be used for analysis and whether they were willing to be interviewed.

The level of agreement to participate was in all cases very high. The students seemed to appreciate the efforts of their teachers to improve the quality of their courses, so generally saw themselves as willing participants and partners in the venture. The fact that feedback was translated into visible improvements definitely helped in encouraging students to make time available to provide the information. We noticed a distinct contrast in the students' attitude to that towards a compulsory student feedback questionnaire scheme which was introduced at the same time. The requirement to complete questionnaires every semester has become widely viewed as a ritual chore because the feedback is not visibly sought by the faculty themselves and impacts on teaching have rarely been noticed.

The researchers also dealt carefully with potential conflicts between assessment and the introduction of journal writing and other innovations. In some cases the journals made no contribution to the students' grades.

The nursing course is used as an illustration of how the issue was handled when journal writing was assessed. Initial journals were not graded for assessment. These journals were mainly used as documentation of learning progress, so that students themselves could review their own learning, and share the learning with peers and teachers. The final paper submitted at the end of the semester was graded. The grading criteria were based on the student's progress, their ability to critically analyse the issues and their fulfilment of general academic expectations such as clear expression of thoughts and correct referencing of material.

The students were reassured that the grades they attained would not be associated with the outcomes of any use of the journals for evaluation purposes within the research project. Such an association was in fact not possible since the grades were submitted at the end of the academic year, before the research team even examined the journals seriously. The students were also assured that confidentiality and anonymity of individual identity would be protected. Participation in the study was voluntary. Students had the right to ask not to be included in the study and their journals would then not be included in the analysis. These students would not be penalised in any way. All students agreed to contribute their journals to the research.

The research setting and the courses examined

To understand the context of the study, it is necessary to provide some background regarding recent associated developments within the university and the public healthcare system. These developments have reflected on the courses included in the study, the details and teaching formats of which are given. Each of the five courses is offered for the development of professionals for allied healthcare fields. Each of the programmes contains an element of professional clinical practice.

The university was first established as a technical college and was upgraded to polytechnic status in 1972. The majority of programmes offered by the polytechnic were vocational in nature and largely followed the technical-rational model described by Schön (1987). The model was evident in that programmes largely followed a behavioural objectives approach. This format aims to describe all learning outcomes for a course or programme. Teaching focuses entirely on directly measurable goals with a consequent loss of spontaneity, and instead promotes a mechanical, peda-gogical format. Atkin as early as 1968 described the danger in this format as leading to lost opportunities when the tea-cher's attention is focused on a few behavioural goals that provide limits to the range and context of learning. Fish, Twinn and Purr (1990) contend that in the technical-rational model, professional expertise was considered a less presti-gious element of programmes where professional status was defined in terms of theoretical or 'intellectual' knowledge assessed by formal examinations.

Professional practical expertise was relegated to separate assessment by practical examination. This was evident in programmes offered by the polytechnic in the manner in which clinical practice was managed compared to the related theoretical components, the lack of resources provided by the polytechnic and the level or lack of responsibility assumed by the clinical departments.

During the late 1980s the number of undergraduate and postgraduate degrees being offered by the polytechnic increased significantly and the institution started the development towards attaining university status. A part of this move included increased levels of internal quality assurance that placed a greater emphasis on the quality of teaching and learning. The programmes included here were developed or upgraded as a result of this progress. They were then validated in the period immediately preceding the institution being granted university, and consequently self accreditation status, in late 1994.

Parallel to the developments in the tertiary sector, the public healthcare system also went through a period of considerable change. Prior to 1990, the government controlled the public healthcare system but in December of that year the Hospital Authority was established to manage all public hospitals in Hong Kong. A major development with this change, was the commitment of the Hospital Authority to developing a patient-centred healthcare system.

Fish, Twinn and Purr (1990) discuss the situation where professionalism has, in the past, been used as the excuse for clinging to unquestioned tradition, routine and repetitive practice. The description resonates in this study's setting both in the education and practice of healthcare professionals. The initiative taken with the setting up of the Hospital Authority and the developmental changes at the university have encouraged the shift towards the goal of developing insightful practice, professional judgement and continuous refinement of practice. This has influenced and strengthened the need to develop student-centred learning, with an emphasis on developing reflective practitioners.

The reflective practitioner model of education, Fish, Twinn and Purr (1990) suggest, encourages the notion of reflection beyond that of critical self-appraisal and problem solving, and necessitates the creation of a learning environment that in all parts encourages a way of learning through practice. Within the reflective practitioner model it is important to develop the student's ability to understand and appreciate the concept of artistry which allows competent professionals to handle the indeterminate areas of practice (Schön, 1987). This 'artistry' is more than the knowledge, skills and attitudes considered important for a professional group; it must also include the knowing-in-practice that allows professionals to make sense of individual practice situations (Fish, Twinn and Purr, 1990).

The remainder of this chapter gives more specific details about the five courses examined in this study. These courses are summarized in Table 2.1. The term 'course' is, of necessity, used rather loosely. The first two courses referred

Table 2.1 A summary of the five courses.

Target group	Post experience nurses	Clinical educators	Physiotherapy	Occupational Therapy	Radiography – first phase	Radiography – second phase
Program level	BSc	PgD and MSc	BSc	BSc	BSc	BSc
Type of students	registered nurses	post-experience clinical practitioners	undergraduates	undergraduates	undergraduates	undergraduates
Mode	part-time	part-time	full-time	full-time	full-time	full-time
Number of students	79	6 and 30	160 (in 2 years)	100 (including 2 years)	70 second year students	70 second year students
Number of staff/facilitators	3	3	6 lecturers and 3 clinical supervisors	2	6	1
Length of module/subject	1 subject in a 2-year course	14 weeks (1 semester in 2 years study)	12 weeks	1 semester	2nd year in a 3-year course	1 semester
Frequency of sessions	4	1/week	weekly meeting	weekly tutorial	4 per course	1 per week
Focus of reflection	contemporary nursing issues	clinical teaching, experiential	client management and learning contract	clinical visit and class activity	clinical experiences	relating theory to clinical experience
Method of journal keeping	journal submission at regular intervals, 4 journal entries and final paper submitted	weekly entry in logbook	tape record or write in logbook before, during and after the clinical placements	write on a specific topic after several meetings	reflection before, during and after each clinical placement	reflective journal – personal
Frequency of sharing journal entries	4 sharings	once per week	aim to have short weekly sessions	two feedback sessions in a semester	during and after clinical blocks	1–3 students per week. Each student once or twice
Time allocated to reflection discussion	2 (hours) × 4 (sharings) = 8 hours	1.5 hours per session	about 30 minutes per session	2 hours per session	1 hour per session	10–20 minutes per tutorial
Tape recording of sessions	yes	yes	no	no	no	no

to below are discrete ones within a degree programme. The remainder refer to elements within degree programmes, mainly associated with the clinical practice component, though not necessarily constituting a specific course in the university handbook.

Post-experience nurses

The research was introduced among the first year students of the part-time post-registration degree programme. A subject *Nursing I: Basic and Dynamics* adopted the reflection-in-action approach intended to promote awareness and critical analysis of professional issues among the students. The students were experienced registered nurses with an average of nine years of clinical experience in various fields, bringing with this experience a reservoir for reflective learning.

Clinical educators

A course for clinical educators was mounted using a reflective teaching and learning approach. The 14-week clinical educators' course entitled, *Clinical Education Techniques*, followed a specific syllabus, set of objectives and assessment. To cover the syllabus, appropriate handouts and reading materials were provided for each section to be covered. The participants were asked to keep a reflective journal, to write something about a subject of interest from their reading or from their daily work experiences which was relevant to both clinical education and the topics covered in the syllabus. They were requested to report back to the group at least one item from their reflective journals each week. This course has now been offered four times.

Physiotherapy undergraduate students

Third year physiotherapy students were prepared for reflection during clinical placements through class discussions. The discussion was centred on how to develop reflective strategies which would promote critical thinking and clinical reasoning. However the plan for keeping reflective diaries raised little interest among the students. The main reason given was that it was too time-consuming. Discussion with the few interested clinical educators and lecturers concluded with a modification to 'pure' journal writing. Reflection on the learning-teaching process could use learning contracts as the basis for reflective learning. The clinical educators and

lecturers were all involved in this tripartite approach. During
clinical placements, the students drew up learning contracts
and discussed them with the clinical educators. Throughout
the placement, the three parties concerned reflected on the
progress of the learning contracts in the form of tape
recordings.

Radiography undergraduate students

The groups taking part were second year BSc students.
Reflective practice is encouraged as one of the measures to
ensure students receive an academically challenging and
vocationally relevant education, in line with the stated programme aims, and so a student centred learning approach is
encouraged.

Clinical blocks follow distinct periods of theoretical
development at the university and the placements a student
will attend during each block are directly related to the theory that has been covered. The first phase of the intervention
was aimed at encouraging students to reflect on the progress
they were making in the clinical setting. The second phase
focused on an academic subject and was aimed at encouraging students to reflect upon, and use their clinical experience
to develop understanding of issues relating to patient
management.

Occupational therapy undergraduate students

The study centred on the first year students of the BSc degree
in occupational therapy. Students undertaking the subject
Introduction to Occupational Therapy were required to
write reflective journal entries about class activities and
clinical visits engaged in during their first semester on the
course. Learning activities were utilised to facilitate students
to develop a professional attitude and to understand the
underlying concepts and principles of occupational therapy.

Part II
Developing reflective teaching in five healthcare courses

Chapter 3
The action research process

Frances Kam Yuet Wong, Alice Yuen Loke and
Marian Wai Lin Wong

Introduction

This chapter discusses the experience of promoting reflective
practitioners in nursing, using the action research approach.
Although the group of students were nurses, the principles
generated from the action research can be applied across
different settings, particularly in the education of healthcare
professionals.

The notion of promoting reflection as a learning strategy
was introduced to a group of nursing students who were
returning to university to study for a degree. As mature part-
time students they would all have developed a significant
experience base and were currently working as nurses. The
subject involved was *Nursing: Basics and Dynamics*, the aim
of which was to facilitate the re-examination by students of
the value of nursing in the changing healthcare environment.
It was thought that this aim might not be easy to achieve
because these students were experienced nurses who were
usually considered to possess a preconceived set of values
about the profession. However, their experiences provided a
rich resource for further learning. A search of the literature
indicated that reflection embodied particular features that
appeared to be useful in helping address the course aim, and
also that reflection is regarded as a valuable learning strategy
in the education of health professionals.

It was found that first, reflection enhances the integration
of theory and practice (Leino-Kilpi, 1990; Saylor, 1990;
Atkins & Murphy, 1993; McCaugherty, 1991a; Snowball,
Ross & Murphy, 1994). Second, it helps the students to
examine alternative ways in dealing with problems; and
third, it facilitates a re-visitation by students of their experience and a viewing of the world in a different perspective
(Boud, Keogh & Walker, 1985; Mezirow & Associates,

1990; Wong, Kember, Cheung & Yan, 1995). These learning outcomes are of particular importance to the education of professionals because the real-world practice that the practitioners encounter each day is dynamic and varied. The practitioners need to take account of the contextual variables in each human interaction and come up with clinical solutions that suit individual client needs (Argyris, Putman & Smith, 1985; Schön, 1987). It was felt that reflection would help students achieve a higher level of learning.

However, reflection was a new concept to both the teaching team and the students. A number of questions emerged as the curriculum was being planned. These included:

- What are the best strategies to facilitate reflective learning and teaching?
- How should reflective learning be monitored?
- How do the teaching team know that the strategies are effective?

To address these questions, we considered both the conventional research approach and the action research approach. The conventional research approach normally involves the comparison of two groups: the group undergoing reflective learning and the group receiving regular teaching. The effects of learning are then evaluated at pre-specified points of time. We found this approach to be somewhat mechanical and the division of the class into two groups defeated the original teaching goal of promoting reflective learning. There was enough literature suggesting that reflective learning was a commendable strategy to prepare practitioners who could deal with the reality. We were not interested in comparing the effects of reflective and non-reflective learning but were rather eager to explore the best ways to facilitate reflective learning. We then decided to adopt an action research approach to tackle the issues at hand, i.e. how to effectively facilitate reflective learning, and how to monitor and improve the teaching-learning process. The obvious starting point of the endeavour was to determine what action research involved.

What is action research?

The definition provided by Kemmis & McTaggart (1982, p. 5) proved to be a rather useful guide. They stated that:

'Action research is a form of collective self-reflective inquiry undertaken by participants in social situations in order to improve the rationality and justice of their own social or educational practices, as well as their under-standing of these practices and the situations in which these practices are carried out.'

Kemmis & McTaggart further elaborated that action research is composed of a series of cycles. Each of the cycles consists of a spiral of steps which include planning, action, the evaluation of and reflection upon the outcome of the action.

The logic governing action research, resembles that of reflection. Schartz (1993) argued that action research is not merely a method but a way of reflection on teaching which creates an inquiry culture in education. Action research is a conscious and deliberate approach to analyse information in the practice situation. It should ultimately lead to strategic action based upon the rational analysis of the results (Tripp, 1990). Learning and improvements to the existing situations occur through the iterative or cyclical processes (Kember & Kelly, 1993). In the education setting, action research is a 'researching while teaching approach' (Schartz, 1993). Teachers research the teaching situation, and improve teaching and learning based upon the information collected from the research process. Action research is a method of inquiry, which can help to bridge the gap between theory, research and practice in education (Holter & Schwartz-Barcott, 1993).

Preparation for the action research

The action research took place with the first year students of the post-registration degree programme at the Hong Kong Polytechnic University. After studying the literature, we decided that an action research strategy was the appropriate approach for us to monitor our teaching initiative and to improve upon the process as we progressed. Before the start of the academic year, the teaching team met several times to formulate the teaching plan and the learning strategies for the subject. Journal writing and dialogue were employed as the essential learning activities because, as demonstrated in the literature, these learning approaches are conducive to reflective learning. Journal writing can stimulate thinking (Richardson & Maltby, 1995) and it also encourages the elaboration of the thinking process through words (Yinger & Clark, 1981), while dialogue facilitates reflective conversation among students (Saylor, 1990). For the teachers, journal writing is a useful document to monitor the presence or absence of reflective thinking among students (Wong, Kember, Chung &Yan, 1995).

The mechanism for monitoring the action research project was also developed before the actual implementation of the subject. We decided to collect data from different sources, which included observations, interviews, student journals and teacher reflection, and to take notes on the observation made during the student dialogue sessions. The aim was to document the progress of student learning. Plans were made to interview a number of students during and at the end of the semester to explore their interpretation and practice of reflection as well as suggestions for further curriculum development. Independent research assistants who were not part of the teaching team were to conduct the interviews. This arrangement aimed at facilitating free expression by the students in the interviews.

The students were scheduled to submit four journals and a final reflective paper four to six weeks apart throughout the academic year. Dialogue sessions were arranged on the same day as the journals were due. The students could then share their journals with each other. The interim journals were not graded but students needed to submit a final reflective paper at the end of the academic year as part of the assessment. We would read the reflective papers and monitor the development of reflective learning of the individual students. We held weekly meetings to discuss the progress of the students and the information collected from observations, journals and interviews. As a result, we could modify our plans to address students' learning needs without having to wait until the end of the academic year which is usually too late to make changes.

The process of the action research

At the beginning of the action research, we believed that our plan was well conceived and a major change to the curriculum plan seemed not necessary. As we implemented the plan, collected information and progress was evaluated and reflected upon, it was found that the students were not responding well to the learning arrangement especially at the beginning of the academic year. They seemed to have difficulty in mastering the essence of reflective learning. We felt that it was necessary to make major changes to the original plan. The process included going through three cycles of the plan-action-evaluation-reflection action research spiral. The duration of each cycle happened to be evenly distributed throughout the year, each lasting about eight weeks. Table 3.1 provides a synopsis of the process. Details of each of the cycles are presented in the following sections.

Table 3.1 Cycles of the action research process.

	Teachers' revised plan of teaching	Observation of student's reflective learning
First cycle		• very descriptive journals • little development of perspectives • weak integration of knowledge and practice • students expressed boredom in dialogue session and journal writing • sought direction and stimulation
Second cycle	• reinforce the use of work episodes for reflection focusing on one theme • use combined group dialogue instead of small group dialogue to stimulate ideas	• combined group dialogue provided students with opportunities to review and organise thoughts and insights • some students took a broader perspective in viewing the issues, and were able to identify different factors affecting the issue • theory-practice gap still prevailed
Third cycle	• arrange discussion of exemplar cases from their students' own discussion groups • teachers to work through the reflective process with students	• students began to have a better appreciation of what reflection meant • seemed to have gained confidence in validating their own reflective process

The first cycle

In the first cycle, the students underwent three small group dialogue sessions and submitted two journals. The journals submitted at this stage were descriptive and demonstrated little development of reflection, the students failing to capture their work experiences and reflect upon them. Very often, they just wrote a superficial account of a clinical incident. Some students made an effort to search related literature but they were not able to utilise it to shed light on their practical encounters. It was observed in the dialogue sessions that the students were repeating themes and they expressed boredom in the discussion. They were searching for direction and stimulation. The students interviewed at this stage said that they did not feel the course was helping them to learn. There were demands for clearer guidelines and model answers to follow in writing the journals. One student said in the interview:

'I found that writing the journals were very difficult. Maybe I am still not familiar with the learning style in tertiary education. Lecturers gave us some very simple guidelines. We didn't have any idea on the content ... it is impossible for us if the lecturers do not give us more standard guidelines. It would be better to get more materials from past students.'

The second cycle

The second cycle began when the teachers reflected upon the students' learning development in the first cycle. The teachers identified the need to foster reflective learning among students with alternative strategies. Students were reminded to make better use of their daily work encounters for reflection. The small discussion groups were brought together in a large peer group discussion to stimulate thoughts and generate richer discussion. This arrangement seemed to achieve two outcomes. First, students had the opportunity to consolidate their previous discussions and to re-organise their ideas so that they could present their thoughts clearly to classmates. Second, the large class took an outsider perspective and could offer opinions which were different from the small group. In the interview, when asked about the impact of this intergroup discussion, students said that they had new ideas after hearing comments from classmates.

Some students were stimulated to re-examine their past clinical practice, as one student elaborated during an interview in the second cycle:

'In the past, I spent a lot of time taking notes without any time to think about it. I regarded what the teacher told us as absolute truth because s/he was an expert. But after I had learned to reflect, I began to reflect on what our lecturer told us. For example, I used to report to the doctor when a patient complained of pain. Now I'll examine him first. It's different from my usual practice. I used to report to my senior or doctor and then I wrote it down on the records. Now I begin to ask why our lecturers taught us to do so. I ask myself what kind of treatment did the doctor give? Did the doctor give the right treatment to the patient?'

Although the students began to use their real life clinical experiences in the learning process, the analysis was not critical enough. The teachers observed that there was a common phenomenon, which we called the 'bikini phenomenon'. The students would write about a clinical incident in relation to the professional theme and then they would follow this by writing what should be done as suggested in the textbook. The descriptions were presented as two distinct pieces of discussion. The students were not able to identify the crux of the matter, or to use the literature to help support their points of view when exploring an issue. For instance, a student would write about a non-compliant patient, suggesting that the non-compliant health behaviour might be a consequence of the psychological and social states of the patient. The student, in the same journal, ended with an authoritative declaration emphasising the importance of the nurse's role in health education to promote health behaviours. This is a typical case of the bikini phenomenon when the students failed to relate the practical incident to textbook knowledge. The effect of health education on the compliance of health behaviour obviously needed to be tested but the relationship between the two was taken for granted by the student. Although the student suggested that the non-compliant behaviour was related to multiple factors, she unfortunately failed to question the absolute value of health education. The teaching team felt that there was a need to introduce further measures to help students be more critical in their reflection.

The third cycle

In the third cycle, the teachers chose some of the exemplars for discussion with the students from case histories. These cases were selected from the student members who demonstrated reflection. There were one or two such students in each group of eight. The selected students would work through the cases with their peers and explain the reflective process involved. The students began to have a better appreciation of what reflection meant and gained confidence in validating their own reflective process. A student gave the following account in an interview when asked about the effect of group dialogue:

> 'Small group discussion helped me a lot. They [other classmates] are from different hospitals, different wards. Sometimes, they talked about their experiences, which I have never heard before. They shared their experiences and practices. I can remind myself what to do when I face similar situations. Reflective learning is like a light bulb in my mind; it will switch on suddenly.'

The students acknowledged that the combination of group discussion and journal writing helped them compare different viewpoints and repeatedly think through situations. The outcome of critical reflection often resulted in a transformed perspective and action. One student said:

> 'I used to treat patients from a nurse's point of view. Sometimes it was quite routine and institutionalised. In fact individual care has always been mentioned but we used to do work for our own convenience. Now we try to meet the patient's need. For example, I once saw my senior directly condemn those mothers as lazy who were unwilling to do postnatal exercises. At the time I didn't think there was anything wrong with the senior nurse. But now I realise that it was a personal attack. After I took this course I realised that every person has his/her own character and we have to respect individual choices. We need to tell the patients the possible outcomes without too much personal prejudice, and let the patients themselves choose.'

At the end of the subject, we classified the students' journals into three categories using the coding scheme suggested by Wong, Kember, Chung & Yan (1995) which is actually a preliminary model developed from the Mezirow & Associates (1990) model. Simply put, there were three categories, the non-reflectors, reflectors and critical reflectors. The non-reflectors were those who were very descriptive in their journals and made no effort to integrate prior knowledge with new appreciation. The reflectors were those who could identify relationships between prior knowledge and new knowledge and arrive at insights. The critical reflectors were those who constantly referred to their practical experience, validated the taken-for-granted assumptions and were able to attain transformation of perspective.

About two-thirds of the students achieved some outcome from reflective learning. There were still one-third of the students who were not classed as reflectors. These students still passed the subject because, according to the traditional academic view, they provided evidence of satisfactory learning, for example many of these students had submitted a reasonable literature review on the topic. However they failed to personalise their learning through reflection. These students usually maintained their original worldview, and seldom questioned the points of view presented in the text-book. They regarded the textbook as a source of authority.

It is not surprising to see that about one-third of the students were regarded as non-reflectors despite all the efforts made to foster reflection. Reflection involves the students in making conceptual changes. It meant that the students needed to conceptualise the world in a different way. In doing so, they needed to challenge the routine and taken-for-granted practices. It was not easy, particularly for the students in this study who were all experienced nurses. The attempt to change one's deeply held values through the educational process requires continuous effort. The effects of an attempt in just one subject (as was the case in this study) to contribute to the continuing development of the students, are not always seen immediately.

Learning from the action research

This action research project has contributed to improvement both in the educational process and in the learning outcomes. The process of the action research itself has fostered in teachers their own development as researchers and reflective teachers. The project demonstrates how a new concept in teaching and learning can be introduced. The experiences show clearly that initial plans rarely work precisely as expected and therefore there is need for evaluation and refinement.

Teachers as researchers and reflective practitioners

With the advances in learning technology, the role of the teacher is undergoing rapid change. Teachers cannot survive by simply being agents for the transmission of knowledge. A vast amount of information is now available in different modes such as books, electronic media and world wide web sites. Teachers are perhaps gradually becoming the least effective and least efficient instruments in delivering information. Teachers today are required to be facilitators of a conducive learning environment and not just to be seen in the traditional role of transferring knowledge to students. They must function as engineers of curriculum construction and facilitators of a learning environment that is responsive to the dynamics of students' needs. The new generation of teachers are those who are willing to introduce innovative measures of learning and teaching and be challenged to help students achieve higher levels of learning. In the process of implementing these new measures, teachers need to monitor and evaluate the process, and make improvements based on evidence. In this respect, innovative teachers will benefit from being researchers as well. At the same time, the teachers need to be reflective so that they can modify the curriculum in light of the students' responses.

The experience in this action research project is that not only have students learned from the subject, but we also have learned from a project in which the students have played a key role. Close monitoring of the students' progress in reflective learning was important so that appropriate measures could be introduced immediately. In this situation, teachers need to engage in reflection as vigorously as we would require of the students. Having certain attitudes, as revealed by Dewey (1933), was essential to students and teachers alike if they were to get the most out of the reflective learning and teaching experience. These attitudes include open mindedness, a sense of responsibility and a wholehearted approach.

- Open-mindedness is an active desire to give consideration to the facts from whatever source they originate and to give full attention to alternative possibilities. Individuals who have an open mind are willing to question their own views.
- Being responsible is a desire to synthesise diverse ideas, to make sense out of apparent non-sense and to apply information in the desired direction.
- Wholeheartedness gives individuals the internal strength necessary for genuine reflection. It enables the individuals to work through their fears of making mistakes and insecurities of being criticised. It gives one the courage to analyse and evaluate the experience and oneself.

These three attitudes existed among reflective students and were particularly prominent among the critical reflectors. Being equipped with these attitudes was of value when attempting to make the action research a fruitful experience.

Promoting the concept of reflection in learning

When we first planned to introduce the concept of reflective learning in the curriculum, we were not certain if the plans would work, although we were optimistic. However, our optimism did not last long. A few weeks after the start of the term, the students expressed insecurity in their learning and were demanding prescriptive guidelines in writing the journals. We acknowledged the anxiety of the students and searched for ways to help them. There were no prescriptive ways to achieve reflective learning since the manner of developing reflective learning is unique to the person. The students can only learn from the world that is constructed and re-constructed by them. A re-conceptualisation of the world does not come from the objective world but rather from the subjective self interacting with the world.

For instance, nurses often regard one of their key roles to be health educators. One student at the beginning of her journal was very confident about her influence on patients' health behaviours through her strategic use of health education. In her subsequent journals, she realised that the clients had their own traditional cultural beliefs of health and illness. At the same time, the nurse's perceptions of health and illness were also influenced by his/her cultural background. The difference between nurses and the patients is that in their professional preparation, nurses are socialised in the ways of western medicine. This student appeared to be very authoritative in her first journal when she asserted that nurses should educate the clients to conform to a prescribed set of health behaviours. Only after a series of reflective journal writings and dialogues did she recognise that nurses and clients should be mutually engaged in the identification of health goals since health behaviours are governed by contextual variables outside of the health education environment.

This example demonstrates that the attainment of reflective learning is developmental. It needs the teacher's guidance throughout the learning process. The action research process provides the teacher with the opportunity to continuously examine his/her own practice as well as that of the students' responses before making appropriate changes. This is different from conventional teaching when students will usually only learn about the achievement of their learning outcomes at the end of the academic year when it is too late to make changes.

Conclusion

Action research is an effective strategy to engage in new teaching approaches and to monitor their effects. It is designed specifically to bridge the gap between theory, research and practice. Action research incorporates both humanistic and naturalistic scientific methods (Holter & Schwartz-Barcott, 1993). It provides evidence to guide practice and support good practices. However, it is different from the conventional paradigm of research as it concerns doing research with, rather than on people. It is a co-operative effort between teachers and students to chart new paths in education. Since action research is a collaborative effort, it demands the participation and commitment of all involved. At the same time, there is a strong sense of own-ership by members of the project but this also implies the involvement of considerable time and energy. Individuals who undertake action research need to be prepared for the amount of human resources required. The teachers need to be directly involved; they cannot be replaced by others, such as research assistants, who are not part of the teaching team. Another key element in the action research approach con-cerns the personal and interpersonal skills of the teachers/researchers (Meyer, 1993).

The ultimate goal of action research is to improve practice. In the educational context, it is important that both the teachers and students benefit from the process. The con-tinued improvement and testing of innovative measures in teaching and learning remains a challenge to the teachers in the twenty-first century. This century will see a continuation in the explosion of knowledge and advances in technology. For teachers to succeed in this rapidly changing world, they need to grow with the students. Such growth can be achieved by engaging in action research that fosters in teachers their development as researchers and reflective practitioners. The beauty of action research is that the teacher and students work collaboratively, exploring new approaches in teaching and learning, and made further improvements to enhance better learning in the future.

Chapter 4
Integrating theory and practice

Jan McKay

Introduction

This chapter discusses an intervention that was aimed at encouraging radiography students to take greater responsibility both for their learning and their understanding of the relationship between theoretical learning and its application in clinical placements.

Traditionally, the predominant model of professional education has been that described by Schön (1983) as 'technical rationality' which emphasises the teaching of technical expertise and systematic procedures. This is the model which, until relatively recently, has predominated in radiography education. Periods of theoretical learning, mainly the transmission of theory through lectures, would be followed by a clinical placement. Frequently, little or no effort was made to link theory with clinical practice.

When the radiography programme at the Hong Kong Polytechnic University was upgraded from diploma to undergraduate degree, the programme team determined to develop the teaching and clinical programme so that it was student centred. The pattern of development of individual courses is now very different from the traditional structure described above. The number of lectures has been reduced and the use of practical/laboratory and tutorial classes widely developed. Material within subject areas has been rationalised so that students can expect to undertake background reading for specified topics where the learning is factual and well explained in texts. The development of courses throughout the programme is designed to encourage integration between courses and years in the programme. An effort has been made to make the style of teaching/learning relevant to the intended outcomes. The aim has been to develop a graduate who can be regarded as an 'advanced beginner' according to the model suggested by Benner

(1984), i.e. someone who can demonstrate marginally acceptable clinical performance having coped with real situations or had them pointed out by a mentor. At the same time they are expected to have developed the independent learning skills required to remain current within a rapidly evolving profession.

The intervention comprised two phases, each consisting of two cycles of action. The inter-relationship between the cycles is illustrated in Table 4.1. The participants were second year students who already had some clinical experience. Clinical education placements were included as discrete blocks throughout the programme, designed to provide students with actual experience in the areas they had been developing in their theoretical courses.

Encouraging students to acknowledge their own progress – Phase A

The aim of the first phase was to encourage students to become more aware of, and to reflect upon, the progress they were making in their clinical placements in terms of meeting the objectives set for the current block of clinical experience.

Table 4.1   The inter-relationship between the cycles in the programme

Phase/action cycle	Form of intervention	Changes incorporated for next cycle
Phase A Cycle one	Students provided with structured reflective journal for reviewing and reflecting on progress in meeting clinical experience objectives	Format of journal restructured to provide a more open response from students
Cycle two	Students provided with revised, semi-structured reflective journal for reviewing and reflecting on progress in meeting clinical experience objectives	Clinical experience used to inform class room learning
Phase B Cycle three	Students encouraged to keep reflective journal and use clinical experience to inform tutorial discussions. Contributions to discussion voluntary.	Contributions mainly voluntary but students could be selected if response was low, and/or they had not contributed previously.
Cycle four	Students encouraged to keep reflective journal and use clinical experience to inform tutorial discussions, as for cycle three.	

Cycle one

The students were asked to keep a structured, reflective journal. Prior to the start of the next clinical block they were encouraged to review the Clinical Studies objectives for the two blocks they had already attended and write in their journal the degree to which they felt they had met the objectives. Areas of accomplishment were to be noted as well as areas they believed required further refinement. They were then asked to review the objectives for the coming clinical block (incorporating two or three placements), make notes about what they would like to achieve from it and to set a goal for each placement they attended.

Rather than stimulating reflection, the provision of objectives reduced most of the students to ticking objectives met and making brief comments on others. A typical, list-like response was given as:

'Objectives not yet achieved:
(1) Arrangement of patient for changing of clothing
(2) Management of children when crying
(3) Setting of exposure factor
(4) Decision of examination according to information on request form'

Cycle two

Reflection on the first round led to revisions being made to the reflective journals for the second round. The journals were divided into sections. Students were asked first of all to review their previous experience in light of the current clinical objectives, then to state what progress they would like to achieve during the course of the clinical block. They then set their own specific objectives and reviewed progress for each individual placement. Finally they made an assessment of overall progress at the completion of the block. The following quotation is typical of those produced from this revised arrangement and clearly shows an advance on the quote given following the first cycle.

'Another problem which is annoying me is exposure factors, I am still not able to grasp the setting of the exposure accurately. I sometimes feel confused about the effect of KVp and mAs on photographic qualities. The unique means to solve the problem is to be clear about the concept of KVp and mAs on film quality. This can be attained by getting more experience. Lastly, as the criteria for a passable film is very subjective, I am not clear whether a film is correctly exposed sometimes.'

Experience from the two cycles of action suggests that an over-structured journal format, as provided for the first cycle, is likely to stifle individual reflection and lead to stereotypic responses. The provision of one or two headings for the second cycle has led to a more reflective response from the students. In a situation such as this where the students were required to reflect on specific topics, a semi-structured format seems to serve a useful purpose.

Programme developments from the first two cycles – outcomes from Phase A

Following these two cycles, with students engaging in and recording individual reflective analyses, it was felt that the separation of the reflective exercise from the more formal clinical assignments reduced the students' concentration on the reflection exercise. Rather than make the reflection exercise additional to the clinical assignments, it was agreed to reformulate the assignments to include more clearly the reflective process.

Reformulating assessments

The first of three major stages of clinical experience was regarded as being the most structured in that it required students to identify discrete areas of information and seemed not to encourage reflective learning. The assignments now require the students to discuss their own ability to perform and assess the outcomes for the examinations and procedures they are analysing.

The second stage required students to produce clinical case studies for each area of clinical experience. Students report on, and discuss, a case that differs for some reason from the normal department procedure. At the third stage the students make a comprehensive analysis of two clinical settings they attend, including their own strengths and weaknesses within the team. These two stages allow students to be more reflective and to integrate and apply learning in the manner desired.

Student feedback

When students return to the university after a period of clinical experience, the initial tutorial period for the related professional course is used for students to raise and discuss issues relating to their recent clinical experience. The clinical assignments are used as a basis for the discussion, and they are encouraged to explore perceived differences between their theoretical learning and clinical experience.

The tutorial discussions are considered to be important for providing an avenue whereby students can raise issues that they may consider will detract from the assessment component of the assignments. The question of whether to assess students' reflections is a vexing one and the solution used for this course was designed, on the one hand, to provide freedom for students to be able to raise issues they may feel were too controversial to put into work for assessment. On the other hand they could feel that they were being 'rewarded' for the effort taken to complete the written requirements of the course. One student discussed the pros and cons of assessment from the clinical assignments:

'If marks are given, we will be more serious and more hard working. Probably we will do more. If marks are not given, it is not saying we do it roughly, I think we will not be so hard working. But if marks are given, it seems to be that it is not so good.

[Why is it not so good?]

It is because you dare not write something unusual. For example, something which is commonly seen and something which is definitely right, and you can ensure you are not going to get wrong. Also I think it's not so good.

I think if marks are given, the things which can be learnt will be less ... The scope is not so wide.'

The concern that students felt if they did not produce work as they saw was expected from their teachers, was an important reason for incorporating feedback tutorials.

'In our placement, we have made modifications to our knowledge and become more informal. A third person might regard it as doing something wrong, but you have actually used and applied the knowledge in practice without being noticed. If you write this in the journal, others might feel uneasy when they read about the techniques being employed. We have to write formal techniques in our written work. The best thing is to have some background support from academic journals.'

The introduction of clinical tutorials at the completion of a clinical block was aimed at providing students with the feedback that is acknowledged as being an important part of the learning process. They were able in this context to raise issues, or discuss experiences that they might not have included in their written assignment for fear of compromising their grades. It allowed them to explore areas of clinical experience that they might not have seen as being different from, or even at odds with what they had learnt in class. This has now been incorporated into the programme as a direct result of the experience gained from the first phase of the study.

Using clinical experience to inform academic development – Phase B

During the course of this project, the regular meetings between members of the study team were useful for informing and prompting actions based on the discussions within the multidisciplinary group. One member noted during a meeting that most of the initiatives being undertaken were aimed at improving the use of reflective learning within clinical settings, with students being encouraged to use their theoretical knowledge to inform clinical experience. It was suggested that clinical practice experience might be equally as effective in informing the development of understanding in the academic setting. This provided the spark for the second initiative introduced into the radiography programme, and composes the third cycle of action.

Cycle three

For one of the courses in the second year of the degree programme, students are expected to develop their own understanding of the issues related to communication and management of patients in the clinical setting. To encourage reflection upon the issues being raised on the course and to encourage integration with the clinical setting, students were asked to keep a reflective journal.

Tutorial classes began with at least one student raising an issue they had noted in their reflective journal. They did not need to raise issues which they felt were too personal but were encouraged to indicate an item they had been reflecting upon. The students were not selected to raise items for discussion but were encouraged to volunteer. The discussions were very wide ranging. Not every student necessarily contributed an item though they were all encouraged to express opinions during the course of the ensuing discussion.

Reflections on clinical experience informing academic learning

At the completion of the course the students were requested to fill out a course review form which asked for their response to four closed questions and four open statements. The aim was to provide feedback related to the students' perceptions of the adequacy of the course in meeting the stated aims and objectives. One of the open statements was: 'I have found keeping a reflective journal has helped/not helped me develop my thinking in this subject/profession.'

The overall response was very positive with 41 of the 57 respondents suggesting that the reflective journal had been useful. Seven gave no answer or were non-committal and nine stated that they did not find it helpful.

There is evidence that students were using their clinical experience when working on the subject, which in turn supported their clinical understanding:

- 'The reflection session at the beginning of the lesson can provide a chance for us to express our feelings about clinical experience. We can raise many ideas and thus try to solve the problem.'

- 'The subject made me think more about the patients' feelings. Even though it was evaluated in the last year in [...] subject, this year this subject made me more aware of it.'

- 'I know more about my patients and why they act like that, ... it is quite interesting because we need to handle such patients. This topic is very useful.'

When asked what aspect they had liked best about the course students gave responses such as:

- 'Tutorial method, the teaching method is open, all the material (majority) comes from the student. The students can share their encountered incidents with the classmates and the teacher can suggest or help to evaluate the incident with the student. It is quite a good way to help the student face the clinical environment. The student interest is raised in this subject.'

- 'Discussion section talking about our clinical experience. It is helpful to discuss patients' response and their psychological needs.'

- 'Discuss and evaluate clinical situations that we have faced in the clinical placements with peers and lecturers – the reflective journals are useful, helping me to identify the correct/incorrect aspects of the case, the dilemma of them.'

Those who did not find the exercise useful tended to suggest that it was a time-consuming effort, or that they did not bother to read it:

- 'Not helped because it is quite time consuming.'

- 'Reflective journal has not helped me to develop my thinking, it is because I do not know what to write down.'

- 'Helpless, I seldom write it and read it.

The students, in general, responded very positively to the incorporation of the reflective journal into the class format, with the overall feeling that they had benefited from the experience. One interesting point was raised by a student who noted:

'Just like keeping a log. One day you'll gain insight on an issue/subject that bothers you. However, it is better to assign at least one student to present his reflective journal for each tutorial.'

Initially, it was planned that the contributions from the journals should be voluntary but this student's comment struck a chord. Not only could students be more encouraged to keep their journals if they knew they were going to be called upon to raise a discussion item but they could also provide support and encouragement for the more reticent members in the group to contribute.

Cycle four

The second time reflective journals were used for this course, the students were informed clearly that they were all expected to make a contribution at some stage, that they would be given the option of volunteering their contribution and a record would be kept of all those who had contributed. A student would be selected if the response was slow, or if there were members who had not previously contributed.

The response to the new format was interesting with only one group out of six requiring intervention to select individuals to raise an item. Even so, when selected, the response indicated that the student had thought about the issues presented. The group dynamics for this one group seemed not to work as well as the others, which may be a contributing factor. There was a concern that those who had spoken up at an early stage may then have felt that they could relax. But the on-going discussion as a consequence of a student's reflection, kept all group members in the discussion process.

There was evidence that the combination of journal writing and discussion resulted in more effective learning outcomes than if the two elements were discrete.

- 'It helps when meeting the patients during the clinical placement.'

- 'I think it can help me to understand more about the real situation and help my thinking in this subject.'

- 'During the tutorial lessons, the reflective journal helps me to analyse, evaluate and solve the problems which I may encounter in the future. It also helps me to know more about the actual condition/position of the Radiodiagnostic Department.'

- 'The students can share their encountered incidents with their classmates, and the teacher can suggest or help to evaluate the incidents with the students. It is quite a good way to help the students face the clinical environment.'

- 'I can know more about the psychological effects in different patients and I can know how to cope with them.'

- 'In the discussions I can share my ideas with others ... to know the patient's response to illness so that I can know what he needs to manage him well.'

Discussion appeared to facilitate greater insights from the journal entries both for the writer and others in the tutorial group.

Overview

The involvement in an action research project has provided an appropriate framework for implementing and refining measures which encourage students to become more reflective. It also has provided positive outcomes.

The concept of actively encouraging reflection and placing it within the formal structure of the courses, has been demonstrated to be an appropriate activity for strengthening the student-centred approach to learning which the programme aims to achieve. The use of reflection has helped break down the traditional barriers between the theoretical and clinical components which are a concern in professional programmes. The students responded positively to the method which encouraged them to use their clinical experience to inform and assist their understanding in a university-based course. This was changed from the initial method which provided a structured format for students to use in reflecting upon their clinical experience. The more formal structure appeared to have been an inhibiting factor in providing a reflective response. The subsequent broadly structured format provided evidence of reflection taking place and led to the redevelopment of the formal assessment elements associated with a period of clinical experience.

The support of the action research team led to the initiation of the second direction taken. The incorporation of reflective journals within the structure of a course, has had positive outcomes. Students were willing to use their clinical experience to help inform their learning on the course and responded well in contributing topics in their respective discussion groups. Some type of demand to raise issues for discussion seemed to have been necessary to encourage the more reticent students but there is no indication that this stifled reflection. Selecting a student to raise an issue when there had not been a ready response from within the group, appeared to make it easier for the more reticent members to contribute, there being no evidence that they were not prepared to contribute. This format is now being pursued as a useful learning tool within other areas of the programme.

The intervention has initiated a more in-depth look at the way in which students can be encouraged to make links between their academic and clinical experiences. It has resulted in a format which is more supportive for the students and which provides a stronger framework in which they can develop their understanding of the overall experience.

The response of the students to the interventions described

here, once again attest to students' positive responses when made equal partners in their own learning process. Working with the students, particularly on the taught course which provides weekly tutorial contact over 14 weeks, it was clear that they wanted to give voice to their opinions and share the concerns and insights encountered along the way.

Chapter 5
The use of learning contracts

Ella Yeung, Alice Jones and Celia Webb

Introduction

The evolution of reflective learning has been an interesting
development over recent years and co-incidentally can be
seen to have paralleled the growth and maturation of the
healthcare profession. In an attempt to facilitate reflection,
learning contracts were adopted as the method of reflective
inquiry for physiotherapy students in their final year clinical
placements. The process of implementing learning contracts
requires the parties concerned to interact in order to enhance
reflective teaching and learning. This chapter discusses the
experience of using learning contracts in the promotion of
reflective learning. The importance of establishing an
appropriate   tripartite   relationship   (student–clinical
educator–university lecturer) is emphasised.

What is a learning contract?

A learning contract can be defined as an agreement about the
type of learning to be undertaken, and is usually negotiated
between two parties, such as a student and clinical educator
(Stephenson & Laycock, 1993). A mature approach to
learning in higher education was described by Knowles
(1983) as essentially a process plan that placed more commitment and responsibility on the student in the teaching-
learning process. It involves students in designing their own
programmes of study, defining the criteria by which that
learning should take place, and engaging in a learning cycle
of planning, monitoring and reviewing how learning is
achieved. It should assist students to adapt their learning to
the different novel circumstances, so often encountered in
clinical practice, thereby giving them confidence in their own
ability and in working with others. However, a strong sense

of collaboration and mutual respect is essential within the framework of negotiated learning (Anderson, Boud & Sampson, 1996). The agreed elements and means of negotiating learning are the tools that enhance the clinical reasoning process and reflective practice which in turn form the basis of effective professional practice (Schön, 1987).

Using this approach, one must ask: How does the student approach the learning process? A learning contract makes explicit what, how and when learning takes place. Writing and negotiating a learning contract is not an easy task for the student or the educator. However, its merit is that the responsibilities involved in professional practice-learning are shared and more clearly defined. Therefore, negotiation or drafting of the learning agreement must involve pro-active responsibilities for both the educator and learner. The initial drafting of the learning contract in itself will assist the student to be better prepared cognitively for the type of learning that should take place during the clinical practicum, as well as for the demands which will be encountered during the particular placement. Furthermore, the flexibility of this approach allows for some re-negotiation of the agreement during the course of the clinical practicum, as deemed necessary through reflections on learning by one or both of the parties concerned.

Implementation of the learning contract

In the physiotherapy undergraduate course, learning contracts were introduced and students and clinical educators encouraged to utilise this approach to learning. Feedback from students and educators has been provided on a voluntary and *ad hoc* basis. As part of an action research programme, a number of students and their clinical educators decided to adopt this approach and participate in a more extensive evaluation of the learning process. This entailed designing and negotiating the learning contract as well as engaging in reflective evaluation by the students, clinical educators and lecturers of the clinical teaching-learning experiences. To clinical educators and curriculum developers, the entire exercise would indicate whether a learning contract was a beneficial adjunct to the conventional teaching-learning methods already established in healthcare education. And despite the often highly structured clinical environment and teaching methods, an examination of how a more flexible approach might assist in the development of more independent, in-depth and reflective learning for the students was still considered relevant. It was considered that the same process was necessary in the development of reflective teaching in educators.

Preparation for the implementation of this approach took the form of sessions where the rationale for the process was explained to, and discussed with, the students and the clinical educators prior to the start of the first block of clinical placements in the final year of the undergraduate degree programme. The learning and teaching approach within clinical education was explained broadly to the students. They were informed that the main aim of the exercise was to discover more meaningful models or processes for improving students' clinical learning. It was made explicit that this action-learning exercise would not be utilised in the assessment of the student. The issue of assessment of a student's performance during the placement, however, did affect the implementation of the action plan, but this will be discussed later.

As an initial introduction and guide to the process, students had been requested to reflect upon their performance in the previous clinical placement. They were asked to review, in detail, the objectives of their placements in the previous year, record in writing those which had been satisfactorily achieved (based on their own perceptions as well as from the comments of clinical educators), and finally, those they thought would require more effort before they could be achieved. It was suggested that as a result of this exercise, students could plan an initial draft of their learning contracts based on the set objectives which they considered to be most relevant to clinical learning for the forthcoming clinical practicum. They were required to state briefly the reasons for the selected goals, as well as the manner and time-frame by which they could be achieved.

Reflection activity schedule

Following the review by the students of their major strengths and weaknesses in clinical studies, they were in a position to begin 'negotiating' contracts with their respective clinical educators. The contract was to include three or four areas in which they wished to improve by the end of the clinical placement. During the placement, the learning objectives could be revised following self-examination by the students and feedback from the educators. Figure 5.1 illustrates the learning contract used by students. Following the drafting of the initial contract, the clinical educator and the lecturer met

From current self evaluation, you have identified areas of:	
Strengths	Weaknesses

Realistic goal(s) to achieve:	How will it/they be achieved	What assistance should I seek?	When do I hope to achieve it/ them?	Comments

Figure 5.1   The learning contract to be used by students

with individual students to discuss and review the content of the contract, clarifying and modifying the objectives to achieve identified goals. They also suggested appropriate ways in which students could be helped to overcome other difficulties. Once agreement was reached, the decision was made about how the student's progress should be reviewed.

The project

Eighteen final year students from three clinical education units, three university lecturers and two clinical educators were involved in the first cycle of the action research project. It was hoped that the learning contract, the reflection activities and their experiences during the clinical placement would allow the students to become increasingly independent and more proficient in clinical decision-making. On completion of the first round of this action-learning plan, some modifications were made for the second round. For example, students and clinical supervisors discussed achievements, problems and means for further progress at more regular and specific intervals as determined by the parties concerned. This action of support by the educational providers was deemed appropriate for ensuring that the contracts would be realistically implemented.

The tripartite relationship

During the development of the learning contract, the three parties (clinical educator–student–lecturer, i.e. the tripartite relationship) met to determine strategies to assist the student's learning and improve areas which were identified as weak or unsatisfactory. The students favoured such a relatively informal and relaxed atmosphere for discussion. It appeared that the focus on the implementation of learning contracts could be shifted towards establishing a stronger relationship between the parties rather than simply fulfilling the objectives of the learning contract within the time schedule.

This tripartite relationship can be viewed as a logical and cohesive approach that brings into fruition the successful education of a competent future practitioner, facilitated by the expertise – and based on the separate strengths – of the clinical educator and the university teacher (Jones, Yeung and Webb, 1998). The strength of the university-based teacher lies in total involvement in, and understanding of, the tertiary educational processes, as well as in their interest in facilitating student learning (Neville & Crossley, 1993). The strength of the clinical educator, on the other hand, is in being well-equipped with all facets of practice skills that are so crucial to professional healthcare practice. If both types of educators' varied skills complement one another in an interdependent relationship, professional education and its corresponding practice is better matched. Therefore, in this tripartite relationship the differences between the two education providers are complementary and of considerable benefit to the students. The spontaneous reflections arising from such collaborative experiences, in turn, provide opportunities for the two educators to modify both their teaching strategies and the content of their respective roles.

The following are comments from the students, lecturer and the clinical educator, demonstrating that the tripartite discussion provided them with a clearer learning direction, allowed more opportunities to clarify misconceptions and resolve differences between university and clinical teaching. It seems that the implementation of this form of communication promotes reflective strategies in clinical learning.

- 'I feel strongly that discussions amongst the three parties were very useful. It appears to be an effective way to convince the students that we [lecturer and clinical educator] are keen to help them. Also it allows opportunity to analyse with the student whether they are heading in the right direction for clinical learning.' (lecturer)

- 'After discussion with him [the student], I discover that he actually wishes to improve his decision making and problem solving skills instead of planning a treatment.' (clinical educator)

- 'It is a useful way to evaluate the progress of the students' performance.' (clinical educator)

- 'It is a good channel for us to discuss and communicate with the clinical educator and the lecturer.' (student)

- 'It is useful to evaluate the progress of the student's performance weekly, as regular evaluation can make the students aware ... I think students can realise their own weak points easier after discussing with others especially the lecturer, the clinical educator and classmates.' (student)

- 'Regular review is a nice idea for the amendment of the learning contract.' (student)

- 'The discussion gave me hints to reflect on my weakness, especially in the way of thinking. I always put things in my mind rather than writing down or verbally presenting the points logically. The clinical educator and lecturer pointed this out and suggested ways to improve such as writing down the points logically before taking any action. It gives me more time to think of what I have thought about and allowed me to eliminate many unnecessary mistakes before taking any action.' (student)

Establishing a learning contract

In the process of arriving at a contract, the students were given plenty of freedom. However it seemed that the students were not comfortable with this or perhaps they were unsure of what was required of them. They seemed to prefer a more directive approach towards completion of the task. Often the guidance of the educator was necessary to assist the students to refine the learning need into specific and achievable objectives. The following examples taken from journal entries and tape recordings illustrate this point.

- 'The first contracts that the students wrote were non-specific and in general impossible to measure. They were asked to re-write the contracts, to make them more specific, and to set targets that would be measurable. The second contracts were written in such a way that they were specific goals that were largely measurable and obtainable within the course of placement.' (lecturer)

- 'I went through their learning contracts. They all expressed their wish, their desire to improve, but these were so vague. They could not identify the area that they wanted to improve. I think they should try to do it step by step, trying to pick out a few areas to focus on and then set achievable goals and try to monitor the progress.' (clinical educator)

- 'There are so many things I want to improve on and I am not quite sure which one is the most important. I wonder if my concerns are in line with the clinical educator's. There were some technical difficulties in setting up a contract. Clinical study is very dynamic in nature. It is difficult to define/measure goals quantitatively. For example, cases can be varied from simple to complicated. What is the evaluative parameter for effectiveness (speed?)?' (student)

Of importance in these examples, was the recognition that the three parties were being stimulated to reflect at this very first stage. Creating opportunities such as this allowed the students to move away from being told what to do towards more experiential learning styles. We recognised that it was important for students to become active in the development of more meaningful understanding of how they learned, and so they were given opportunities to review and clarify the contract.

Clarifying the learning contract

Parsons & Durst (1992) stated that the determining factor in the success of the learning contract is the process of contracting. The contract itself should be viewed as a dynamic and on-going process rather than a static document. The following quotations are typical cases demonstrating the fine-tuning of the objectives.

- 'The student at the beginning states the learning contract. But during the placement, I may identify some special things that I would like them to improve or the things that students would like to improve. I think it is necessary to add this. Take student X, as an example.

Her objectives are very simple, but I find that there are other aspects she should take care of. Although I do not write it down in the contract, I will follow up this aspect.' (clinical educator)

- 'The learning objectives should not be written on the first day the student arrives but when we are familiar with each other. I then know his performance and he knows his strength and weakness so as to develop an appropriate learning contract. It will be more suitable.' (clinical educator)

After drafting the learning contract and through discussion, the student was in a position to review his/her learning needs with the clinical educator. Analysis of the students' weaknesses is no easy task. It was usually triggered by features of the practice situation, identified on the spot and linked immediately to action.

The following example demonstrates how critical reflection is involved in the process of clarifying the learning contract. A student involved in the project indicated that he had difficulty in analysing assessment findings. However, the clinical educator recognised that the student's inability to analyse was due to his poor verbal instruction and his crude assessment skills. So the clinical educator was in a position to discuss with the student and advise him accordingly. Indeed the observation of the student's performance became a stimulus for the clinical educator to reflect critically. This student, with the guidance of the clinical educator, was able to evaluate questions like 'What do I already know?'; 'Where am I now?'; and 'Where do I want to go?'

Negotiating the learning contract

The negotiation between the educators and the students requires openness, mutual respect and trust. However, we found that although we wanted to foster the learning climate by using the contract, the students were hesitant to expose their strengths and weaknesses. The contract was, after all, outcome oriented and there was an assessment component at the completion of the clinical placement. A few examples from the students clearly illustrate this.

- 'Learning contract is a good tool in finding out one's strength and weakness. However, mostly only the weakness is observed rather than the strength. And I guess that not many students dare to state their strength because it may be a weakness in the view of others.'

- 'If the clinical educator is not neutral enough, or is biased against you, after the clinical educator knows your weakness, he will concentrate on this point during the assessment.'

- 'The learning contract will only work effectively if students are honest, and this will only happen in a situation of mutual trust, where areas of improvement are not highlighted as weakness to be put under a microscope for assessment. This is something that needs to continue to be developed.'

Interestingly the clinical educators said that often they did not adhere rigidly to the learning contract but saw it as a tool for better communication. This feeling was shared by the university lecturers as well as the students and led to an intricate tripartite relationship which will be discussed later. The discussion amongst the three parties often assisted in identifying student weaknesses some of which they were not aware of.

- 'Time to focus on their [the students'] specific learning objectives is not easy. The students have patients to treat and my main concern tends to be assisting the students to maximise their learning at that specific time and it frequently does not involve any of their learning objectives. Rather it presents learning opportunities that I do not want the student to miss out ... If an opportunity does arise, then obviously having read the students learning contracts I can assist and give feedback on their performance in achieving that goal.' (lecturer)

- 'The learning contract may not be able to assist students on all different aspects to become a competent physiotherapist ... the student may lack insight into their own problems and therefore be unable to identify their problems and unable to write them down in their learning contract.' (clinical educator)

In some centres, modifications of the learning contract were required after several weeks in the placement. This was an aspect which was important for the students so that they could set their own learning pace and be provided with positive reinforcement when their goals were being achieved.

By using learning contracts, the students became aware of their own improvement and their own learning process. This was another opportunity whereby the students could re-examine their own progress and whether the learning objectives were being achieved. A case study is presented in the Appendix to this chapter to illustrate this.

Carrying out the contract

In one clinical centre, the clinical educator evaluated the students' objectives and rated whether they had reached their learning target by the end of the clinical placement. The criteria for the assessment were based on the aims of clinical placement. The six students were also asked to judge if the contract objectives had been achieved (see Table 5.1).

Table 5.1   Student's and clinical educator's perceptions of the achievement of objectives

Student	No. of objectives set in the contract	Student's perception of the no. of objectives being achieved	Clinical educator's perception of the no. of objectives being achieved
A	4	4	3
B	3	3	3
C	5	5	4
D	4	2	3
E	3	—	1
F	4	2	3

While this table gives very little information about the reflection of the learning experiences, it does provide us with some insight into the achievement of the goals set. The learning contract seems to be an effective teaching/learning strategy when the educators and the students are committed to achieving the objectives by the end of the placement.

As discussed earlier, the process of formulating, clarifying and negotiating the contract allowed the students to reflect upon their own clinical learning in a different way. Comments such as the following were made:

- 'We really recognise our problems through thinking...'

- '... good channel for us to discuss with the clinical educator and the lecturer.'

- 'It is a good way to reflect on one's strength and weakness so as to enhance one's learning.'

- '... know the problem and tackle it exactly.'
- '... allow the students to think the problem closely.'
- 'I think students can realise their own weak parts easier after discussing with others especially the lecturers, the clinical educator, classmates etc.'
- 'It's useful to evaluate the progress of the student's performance weekly as regular evaluation can make the students aware.'

In general the students involved found the learning contract useful if it was used properly. The learning contract allowed them to think about the learning stage they were at and helped them set further targets to achieve.

Evaluation

In healthcare professional training, emphasis is placed on clinical practice which offers an ideal applied learning environment. The therapist must be able to identify the problems of the patient, propose and execute solutions, with continuous evaluation of the effectiveness of the management procedure. Students therefore should be trained to question the assumptions underlying their practice by being motivated, and by analysing and channelling their enthusiasm, as well as by keeping informed of the developments in the profession. In order to assist students to reap the most benefits from clinical practice experiences, educators should evaluate the process and benefits of learning approaches which are different from the traditional technical acquisition of practice skill. It is no longer possible to rely on the conventional teacher-directed, information-giving form of clinical education. The learning contract used in this project serves as a useful model of teaching and learning.

It seems that the extent of the success of the learning contract towards reflective learning in clinical practice will depend very much on the negotiating skills of the students and the clinical educators. Modification of the learning objectives is often necessary as an outcome of reflection on learning strategies. Effective communication between students and educators is essential to assist students in formulating strategies to improve learning. The principal benefit of the contract does not come directly from the contract itself but rather from the communication between the three parties.

With the challenges associated with clinical education, the use of a learning contract seems to be an appropriate tool in the facilitation of the tripartite relationship. By interacting during the process of implementing the contract, all three parties have a commitment to a common ground. The lecturer and the clinical educator may gain insights into how to facilitate the students' learning throughout the clinical experience, and the students are given opportunities to express their feelings. This process could be expected to impact on students' learning. The students see learning more as a process of self-examination and review, rather than purely the acquisition of knowledge and facts. The case study of student M (see Appendix to this chapter) demonstrates that she was made aware of a strategy to enhance her learning outcome. The journal recordings of the clinical educator involved suggested that the learning contract might have exerted an influence on M's learning throughout the clinical placement.

In addition, it was indeed encouraging and reassuring to receive the following comments from the students:

- 'In my previous placements, many students, and even the clinical educator, interpreted the learning contract as "homework" or "duty". Although the students and the clinical educator set the contracts, both parties did not practice them well in the actual learning process. However I recognised the significance of setting a learning contract in this clinical placement. Mr M, the clinical educator, and my lecturer Miss D, allowed me to express my learning objectives without hesitation. They also guided me to incorporate my learning objectives into the whole placement. During the whole placement, Mr M provided feedback on my progress on regular basis. Hence, I could recognise my state of progression. In my opinion, the learning contract was utilised in an appropriate manner in this placement because both the educators and the learners had to put it into "action". I hope other centres could also exercise the same thing.'

- 'In this placement, I feel I have gone some way to achieving the aims in my learning contract. My organisation has been better as I have prepared better in advance and reflected more on the patients' problems and how to best improve their condition. I have also had some good hands on experience and observation of stroke patients, combined with regular discussion. I still have a long long way to go but I feel I have a little more understanding now.'

At the end of the project, it was apparent that the students should be given clearer guidelines when writing the contract. Students do need positive support and guidance from the clinical educator or lecturer to set realistic learning goals and objectives within a placement. There was also a need to reassure the students by reinforcing the fact that the contract must be used to reflect on their learning rather than as measures of their clinical performance.

Conclusion

The experiences described in this chapter suggest that the use of learning contracts can enhance professional practice if the therapists make practice 'more reflective than routine' (Schön, 1987). The process of self-reflection from all three parties should enhance quality student learning in clinical settings. It is imperative that educators provide the opportunities for students to become self-directed, life-long learners. Likewise, it is important that students pursue self-reflection activities that may lead to transformative learning.

Appendix to Chapter 5
Case study of student M

Student M is a final year physiotherapy student who agreed to enter into a learning contract at the beginning of her placement. She stated in her contract that she had difficulty in analysing the findings after examination of a patient and was therefore unable to work out the patient's main problem. Following discussion with the clinical educator and the lecturer, it was identified that student M's problem was due to an inadequate knowledge base and lack of confidence in making decisions about selecting the appropriate treatment modality. In order to achieve this learning objective, student M agreed to:

- read articles and relevant journals relating to the particular medical condition;
- discuss the cases with the clinical educator at least twice a week;
- engage in personal reflection using tape recordings to evaluate her progress, and what helps or hinders her in fulfilling this objective.

The clinical educator and the lecturer agreed to build up M's confidence by:

- giving verbal feedback about whether the analysis was accurate and appropriate during the discussion;
- documenting achievements and positive reinforcement;
- self-reflection and recording how the student progressed in achieving this learning objective.

The following are extracts of the self-reflective diary of the clinical educator about student M through this six-week clinical placement block and gives some insight into the achievement of the learning objective. This can almost be regarded as reflection through recollection (Garman, 1986), i.e. when the clinical educator goes through the four stages of recalling the incident, capturing the incident in tape recording or journal writing, interpretation and confirmation. It is recognised that this process is important for personal and professional development and is regarded as important for examining practice.

Week 1

'Student M is very tense. She shows lack of confidence both in front of me and in front of the patients. She has very weak knowledge base, and inaccurate assessment skills, thus affecting her analysis of the cases and identifying the causes of the patients' problems. Even with a simple joint problem, she needs lots of guidance... Advice was given to her with regards to revision of basic knowledge and the setting up of flow charts to help reasoning and identifying short and long-term goals.'

Week 2

'She has showed some effort to revise and study. However lots of guidance is still needed. She needs lots of time to understand a case. Problem listing has improved slightly. Assessment and treatment techniques have also improved.... I have stopped giving her new cases till she develops better insight into the old cases.'

Week 3

'Still not confident in decision making towards treatment progression. She is too frightened to speak out ... I accompanied her in a treatment session of a shoulder case and guided her all the way through ... No marked improvement this week.'

Week 4

'Still slow in her assessment. Choices of treatment still need guidance. However she is quite comfortable with most of the old cases now ... She is more confident with her presentation.'

Week 5

'Analytical power showed some improvement, she can now work out the main problems of the patient by the end of the third visit of the patient. Still having difficulty with more complicated cases ... Progression of treatment and time management is still a problem. However her presentation skills and confidence level have certainly improved.'

Chapter 6
Writing reflective journals

Kit Sinclair and Harrison Tse

Introduction

This chapter describes the use of journal writing to aid reflection in first year undergraduate students. Journal writing by itself is seen as a valuable stimulus to encourage reflection upon practice (Wagenaar, 1984; Hahnemann, 1986; Bean & Zulich, 1989; Cameron & Mitchell, 1993).

Introducing reflection and reflective journal writing

Occupational therapy undergraduate students were introduced to the use of reflective journals in the subject entitled *Occupational Therapy Theory I* in the first year of their three-year professional education programme. Following specifically designed learning activities and clinical visit observations, students were asked to explain their learning experience in their own words and relate it to their past experience. It was hoped that through the process of reflecting on practical experience and observations, students could gain a better perspective of themselves in relation to their future career. Reflective journal writing was used to assist students to internalise their learning in both cognitive and affective (feelings, attitudes) domains.

During the first tutorial session, discussion took place and handouts were given to students to introduce them to the concept of reflection and the writing of journals. The handout stated that the purpose was '... to develop your understanding of professional knowledge and standards'. A total of 50 students were requested to write reflective journal entries of approximately 500 words for each of six specified class activities and four clinical visits. These activities were listed according to a time schedule given to students on the first day of class. To achieve the task of writing reflective journals, students were asked to explain their learning experience and to comment on any change in perspective or understanding of theoretical principles because of this experience. The following instructions were used to direct students' focus throughout the semester:

'During your *Occupational Theory Theory I* course, you will be involved in various activities and clinical visits. Keep a journal of your feelings and reactions to these activities using a diary style of writing. Focus on an issue that you feel is of particular significance to you. You may use headings and subheadings if desired. Write your diary entries immediately after the activity or visit so that your reactions are fresh in your memory. You can comment later about the same event after you have had time to reflect on it. Write at least one side of one page.'

It was emphasised that the journals should be used by students to monitor their own progress and prepare for the assignment and final examination. They were expected to use journal entries as a basis for contribution to group discussion and feedback on the activity or clinical visit, during which the breadth and depth of learning could be demonstrated. Students could also use the journals as a forum to share problems of learning about concepts and skills related to occupational therapy. To facilitate students' completion of the journal entries with reflection on theoretical issues, guidelines were given to students suggesting that they:

'... briefly describe the experience of learning during the activity. Describe what aspects impressed you most about the activity or visit. Explain your feelings in relation to your strengths, capacities, fears, weaknesses, biases...
... suggest alternative actions you might have taken (or might take next time) to improve the activity or visit and make it a better learning experience for yourself.'

The first cycle

Journal writing was used to facilitate reflection in two dimensions. At the personal dimension, students were expected to write in the journals about their own experience of learning activities. At the group dimension of reflection, students were encouraged to discuss their own experience in the class, as a form of sharing of their personal reflection, from the written journal. Students were asked to submit their journals regularly for comment.

The marked assignment at the end of the course drew on the journal entries. The assignment required students to choose one experience from school or from a clinical visit which was particularly valued as a learning experience and which impacted upon professional development in occupational therapy. From that experience students were asked to write, in about 700 words, a description and some comments about the impact of the experience. This might include the development of understanding, the application of theoretical principles in occupational therapy, the relation to feelings, the evaluation of personal strengths and weaknesses and the change in the students' own perspectives as a result of the experience. This assignment formed the culmination of the work the students had completed during the course. Journal entries formed a basis for the writing of the marked assignment but the students did not receive marks for the entries.

Reflections in the tutor's journal commented on expectations for the level of journal writing:

> 'Initially I did not have high expectations of the students' ability to write reflectively. Being new to the process myself, I was learning along with the students. I collected and recorded the submission of the journal entries but did not mark them or write comments on them. The students seemed somewhat confused about what was required. When this came to my attention, we discussed their concerns in tutorial. I was not able at that stage to give them very clear directions on how to improve their writing since I felt that if I gave them too definitive examples, the students would copy the format directly and not be creative in their own writing.'

About half way through the semester, a tutorial session scheduled for reflective feedback was spent discussing 'reflective learning' and the problems encountered in attempting to write their journals. At this point a handout was prepared and given to students with suggestions about how to improve their reflection. Suggestions included listing their strengths and weaknesses using such sentence starters as 'What I understand well ... What I don't understand or can't make sense of ...'; or 'What went well ... What went badly...'.

The handout also suggested that students attempt to work towards identifying: 'truths you have discovered through your experience'; 'advice to yourself about what to do in the near future'; and 'finding questions which you need to think about or issues which you don't yet fully understand but need to understand'. Copies of some of the more reflective journal entries of their classmates were included to give them examples for comparison. Some of the examples are as follows:

Related to the occupational profile interview assignment:

- 'After the discussion in the tutorial lesson, I discovered that my questions were not broad enough to cover all aspects of my sister's life and I have omitted many details. I hadn't thought that small facts in one's daily life could reflect one's interests. These small facts are useful to our work. They can help us to design the kinds of activities that are suitable for the patients.'

- 'I think when I do a profile next time, I will ask the interviewee some basic questions first (as I did not go deep enough before) because the basic questions can help us analyse his daily life. Then, I will ask him some deeper questions but not too private because if I ask questions which are too private I think he will not answer the questions or will tell lies.'

Related to the clinical visit:

- 'The visit also gives me a positive attitude towards human life. Since, only if people take the initiative to work hard, can an obstacle be removed. Just like these clients who are mentally ill, physically handicapped ... etc; they can live and work like ordinary people after being trained in the skills centre.'

- 'The visit made me understand more about the tasks and roles played by the OT in a skills centre for persons with disability. The most important thing is that I have a chance to make personal contact with people who have physical or psychiatric problems that I have not experienced before. I think I should carry on to actively participate and make contact with these people next time, to be more clear about what are their needs and demands.'

- 'Improvement for next time ... be more relaxed. During this visit, many of us were too nervous, we wanted to make as many notes as possible so that we could get more information for our reports.'

As a result of the mid-term tutorial discussion with students, it was agreed that they would receive specific written feedback on their journal entries giving comments on areas for expansion in reflection.

Evaluation of the first cycle

By the end of the first cycle, the students appeared a great deal more confident in their ability to write reflexively and the improved feedback methods seemed to enhance their reflectivity.

At the end of the course, five students – by the process of simple random selection – were chosen to be interviewed. Conclusions drawn from the interviews were used as a basis for further reflection and for changes made in the second cycle.

Attitude towards journal writing

In general, students found that writing a reflective journal, as opposed to essay or descriptive writing, made a difference to their own learning experience. Of the five interviewees, only one of them reported, when reflecting on the experience in the classroom, that such a difference did not exist. However a difference was found when reflecting on experiences in clinical visits or placements. All the responses of interviewees showed that the nature of such a difference was positive and included cognitive and affective outcomes.

Interviews with the students elicited such points as the need for reinforcement of 'time to think reflectively', to recall incidents and past knowledge, to consider new ideas, to evaluate the learning process and to share it. A student explained this aspect stating:

'Yes, sure. When I am writing the journal, I review the thinking process of the clinical visits. That is, I have seen many psychiatric patients doing light industry tasks. At that time, I wondered why so many patient were doing this. Is that the only training of the OTs? Obviously it's not and raised a question at that time. And when I wrote the journal, I tried to think through the thinking process of this – the question at that time. I linked the knowledge of what I had learnt, and I know for example that we stress the training of the patient's endurance or work habit in the psychiatric field. So, I regard it as the most useful one.'

Another student used the interview opportunity to evaluate the effectiveness of journal writing on his study and learning:

'Yes, [journal writing] will make a difference. Writing the journal after class at least can force me to recall my memory in class. If I did not need to write any journals, I would forget the things from class more quickly. Or it may stimulate me to think about what I have learnt. I think the journal writing can stimulate me to learn something new ... I remembered in one lesson we had a role-play. After the class, we had to write the journal. While I was writing the journal, I was stimulated to think about why I was studying this course. Is it right for me to study in this course? Am I interested? Something like this. These are the questions I have not ever asked myself.... The journal writing helps me think whether I am suited to studying this course.'

Lack of confidence in writing

Some of the students' lack of confidence in writing was reflected in their comments at the end of this first cycle. It was found that difficulties of writing a reflective journal stemmed from:

- the uncertainty about the expectations for journal writing;
- the contrast between experiential and classroom learning;
- the difficulties of language choice and expression.

Uncertainty about expectations

The instructions given to students were described in the previous section. The students seemed uncertain of the expected function, or the ultimate aims, of the journal writing. The following quotation by a student elaborates this point:

'The difficulty I think is that I don't know how to write a journal. That means, I don't know the format of writing journals ... I think the lecturer can help us to know clearly the purpose of the journal and its aim ... I think the lecturer wants to know about our learning process and our attitude, something like that.'

Students commented that they sometimes couldn't find things of interest to write about. Here are two illustrations by students:

- 'Sometimes it's hard for me to get any idea to write or to complete the journal because not everything impresses me.'

- 'Sometimes I found the lesson was not so valuable for me to write in a journal or it is hard for me to recall because I may not do or write the journal after the lesson or I may write it after a week ... In my case, I think I'm a little bit lazy. I think if I am not interested, it was hard for me to write the journal. I think it is no use for me to write the journals just copying from the others and I just write the journals because of the teacher's order. As I have just mentioned, sometimes it may be hard for me to remember because I may write the journal after a week or after a few days or I may find the visit boring or something is not significant for me to write down in the journal.'

Contrast between experiential and classroom learning

The data indicated that students found it easier to write about clinical visits which were concrete experiences and evoked some strong reactions. In contrast, they found writing about issues in classroom learning difficult since they lacked knowledge about the issue, as commented by two students in their comparison between writing about clinical visits and writing about classroom activities.

- 'Well, I find it easy to write a journal on clinical visits because there are many impressions and feelings about the visits ... Well, since we do not have enough time to digest the content from class, even if you write a journal about the [theoretical] issue, you still cannot have a clear understanding of the issue. So writing in the journal is not useful.'

- 'I think it's quite different because I think writing the reflective journal about clinical visits is more useful for us. To recall from memory a typical case on clinical visit and apply the actual situation in occupational therapy, we can use some OT theory or other theory to apply in the actual situation and ask the lecturer. Why do I think [writing about clinical visits] easier? Because when I am in the clinical visit, the event that I face, stimulates me to identify the problems that I don't know. Then it's quite useful for me to write the reflective journal about these problems and ask the lecturer to give some feedback to me about the clinical visit ... Another is I think that year 1 students may not have the basic knowledge to understand the lecture or some notes that they teach us. So, I think that they will not write the reflective journal with so much detail about the problems. The student may not feel the responsibility to reflect all the things to the lecturer.'

Language choice and expression

In some instances, students found it difficult to express themselves in English which is their second language, as suggested by student 2 and 3:

- 'In my case, I think if the journal writing is in English, some times it is difficult for me to express my point of view and ideas.' (student 2)

- 'Some students may not have the review of the lecturer's notes or the content of the lecture and their knowledge is not enough to understand the lecture notes. So, I think they will not reflect the actual points in them that you have to face and [therefore] they will not write in their journals. Also it's difficult for them to use English to explain the difficulties or reflect the actual situation.' (student 3)

Need for more group discussion

Students in general agreed that more group discussion would help the reflective process. Group discussion could also substitute for a degree of individual reflective writing. There was agreement that discussion was fruitful, although they did not always agree on the format of the discussion, e.g. whether lecturers have to be involved.

- 'I think the discussion before the journal writing can stimulate students to remember the lesson content and communicate with classmates about other concepts they have learned. If students have not learned some concepts, then they can exchange ideas and learn more.'

- 'In the case of clinical visits, [individual] journal writing is better, whereas during lectures (and tutorials), it's better to have [group] discussion most probably.'

Conclusions from the first cycle

Changes suggested at the end of the first cycle included a need for a clearer introduction to the importance of reflective journal writing or even having previous students available to discuss the relevance of reflective journal writing to learning, thus adding to the interest and 'excitement'.

Criteria for distinguishing a reflective journal from a non-reflective journal needed to be clarified. Samples of journal writing were seen to be more useful to students after the aim and objectives of journal writing have been given to them, thus deepening their understanding of the values and benefits of the journal writing that they are aiming for and the need to write reflectively. It was also seen that more discussion and feedback was needed to assist the students in their understanding of the process and the content of their writing.

The students' understanding of the meaning of reflection was not restricted to personal reflection but also included the idea of sharing or discussing with others. A number of students commented that they felt more group discussion would help their reflection, before and after journal writing. One student suggested that both formal (in class with the lecturer) and informal discussion (outside class) would be useful. Another suggested that allowing time to write at the very end of class would be best.

In general, most students accepted writing a reflective journal as a requirement of the course. An exception to the positive attitude towards journal writing was reported by a student during his interview at the end of the course. He stated that he was 'forced to review what was learnt', he did 'not think it was useful' and it was regarded as an 'extra task'. Even so, he stated, 'Reflection will help me, but the journal writing will not help me'.

Interviewees repeatedly commented that they reflect more frequently on daily life events than on clinical experience or on classroom learning. By exploring the transfer of the skills in reflecting on daily life events to classroom learning, we may have a better understanding of the conditions for reflection.

Second cycle

The *Occupational Therapy Theory I* course was run the next year for a new group of students. Taking into account the feedback from the previous group of students, more specific guidelines were provided with examples from the previous students' work. At the beginning of the second cycle, the students seemed to be more receptive to journal writing as an activity. This may have been due to the fact that the previous students, now in year two, had shared with them their journal writing experience during informal talks.

As agreed in the evaluation of the first cycle, the journal entries were collected immediately after the activity/visit and students provided with written feedback. Half-way through the programme, a tutorial session was spent gathering feedback and leading discussion with the students about their clinical visits, thus giving them the opportunity to reflect verbally with their classmates on their experiences.

Understanding of expectations

Students in the second cycle seemed to find the reflective writing activity useful. The change of approach at the beginning of the course and the more regular written feedback seemed to have been more effective. They showed a better understanding of the overall aim of journal writing as a tool to learn and construct knowledge from their own experience. The following are some typical examples that show a fairly clear understanding about the instruction of journal writing and its aim.

- 'Actually, it is a reflective journal. We were told to do a mock interview for the case study. We were divided into several groups. Every group received a sheet that showed several situations. We took turns to pretend to be an occupational therapist or a patient. Before we obtained some professional knowledge, we tried to act as an occupational therapist to treat patients. After the lesson, we had to write a journal to think back on what it feels like to be an occupational therapist, or the job of an occupational therapist.'

- 'For a "normal journal", I just focus on the feelings only, say, I like it or I am surprised. But for the "reflective journal", it was quite different. I discovered the weaknesses, advantages and disadvantages from my feelings towards the job. For instance, I can see whether I am suitable for that job from the feeling. It is different from focusing on the feeling alone.'

In general, students regarded the journal writing process as a chance for self-evaluation. This is a typical quotation:

'When you write the journal you know what your weaknesses are. In the future you can make use of it as a reference for self-evaluation. If I had not written the journal I may not have known in what areas I have to improve myself.'

Attitudes toward journal writing

Students also displayed a better attitude towards journal writing. They appeared to take more initiative in writing about activities and feelings.

- 'If I did not write it down, I would just have an impression immediately after the class tutorial [about interviewing techniques] and I might forget it later. However, the journal writing can help me to retain the memory and attitude for making improvements.'

- 'I usually wrote about my feelings at that time. For instance, in an 'interview' role-play, some of us act as patients and some of us act as OT's. It is easier to write about acting as a patient, for example, acting as a lorry driver who has broken some fingers in an accident. We can think of the problems of the patient very easily; say, insufficient financial support, unclear future. However, the one who acts as an OT can hardly think of the solution. The reflection stimulates us to study OT and the way to help the patients solve the problems.'

In response to the suggestions about taking 'on-the-spot notes' in order to stimulate later reflection, the experience of students in this cycle suggested that excessive note-taking can detract from the purpose of the clinical visit. This can be illustrated by the dilemma faced by a student in the second cycle.

'It causes difficulties if you write down too many notes during the "visit". It may even disturb the procedure of the visit or lesson. However, I may get nothing if I don't write down any points! So, the best way is to have a clear mind, and to mark down the basic points and elaborate on them later.'

Similar to the findings of the first cycle, data from the second cycle also showed that the time gap between the happening of an event and journal writing is important for retention.

'The long time gap between the lesson and writing is the difficulty. I sometimes cannot remember at all ... I prefer writing it down right after the lesson or do it on the following day.'

Feelings and reflection

The second cycle of research interviews also focused on the students' writing in the affective domain, providing a better understanding of the relation between feeling and reflection through the dialogue made with interviewees. The following statement was made by a student when asked to elaborate on the relationships between the two constructs.

'It is related to the merit and weaknesses of oneself. If I am a shy person and don't know how to communicate, I may feel miserable during the visit as I find it is difficult for me to communicate with the others. "Miserable" is the feeling. If you write it down in the journal, it is just a "journal" but not a "reflective journal". However, if I can find my weaknesses from the experience of feeling miserable, such as a lack of inherent communication skills and self-confidence, then the reflection of weaknesses and merits can be said to be "reflective".

Data from the interviews suggest that feelings may be a motivation for reflection and help in the retention of an event in long term memory. They can also affect the effectiveness of reflection. The following quotations illustrate this point.

- 'Stronger feelings can help me to learn more. If I have less feeling about something, I will forget it more easily. Feeling can help me to remember things for a longer time.'

- 'I think the usefulness of journal writing depends on the topics being studied. Sometimes, I find journal writing interesting if I think the topic is interesting. However, if the lecturer just taught about the theories, I find it boring. Otherwise, I would treat journal writing the same as composition writing, although it is called a 'learning process', because I was just taught some things but I really don't know what they are. I find nothing to write about if the topic is not interesting.'

Approach to learning

Students appeared to develop an improved learning style though journal writing. Deep learning strategies and the bridge between theory and practice are exemplified in the following quotes.

- 'Before [experiencing journal] writing, I didn't think it would help because it was just like English writing class. You still have to write even if you do not have things to write about. It seemed to focus on writing something that you don't have strong feelings about. However, after the experience of writing, I found that journal writing helped me to think after the visits. I may not have thought about it if I hadn't had to write the journal. The feeling or ideas may have been easily forgotten or missed if I had not thought or organised them. Journal writing can make the segmental things change into systematic ones. It may help me someday when I come across it again.'

- 'New things you see during the visit you may not relate to OT theories. You may just visit it and see what the therapist is doing, but while journal writing, I will refer to what I've learned from lessons. I may find that they did what the theories suggest.'

Language choice and expression

As with the findings of the previous research cycle, it can be seen that language can be a hindrance to reflection. Again, in general, students prefer to use their first language.

'Firstly, it is better to introduce the journal in Chinese. At the beginning of the course, I didn't know what reflection was because I was only given some notes and a sample journal. I didn't know how to write so I did it just like a diary, writing by putting all the data in. As English is not the mother tongue of the students of Hong Kong, it is difficult to be able to do it well in English.'

Students in this cycle seemed to be more comfortable with the style of journal writing. The students' attitude towards language accuracy changed and they tended to shift their attention from the language difficulties they met, to the function of journal writing and putting down their thoughts on paper, as exemplified by the following:

- 'I would recall the feelings and wrote them down at home ... I regarded it as writing a dairy. I could look at them and find out what I'd learnt.'

- 'English. Hmm ... Perhaps because Mrs [...] knows Chinese, I sometimes dare to take the risk of writing wrong grammar. I don't mind if the grammar may not be correct as I think she may understand, but other foreign lecturers may not understand.'

- 'As I've said, written work helps the organisation. Sometimes, we want to share the feelings even though we can't express them well in English.'

Relations between journal writing and discussion

The data gathered from both the first and the second cycle suggested the possibility of using discussion as adjunct to or a substitute for reflective journal writing. In the first cycle, journal writing was found to be an effective learning activity to prepare students for discussion. Research suggested that discussion of reflective writing could add a further dimension to the experience. Critical discourse may serve to develop collective understanding (Carr & Kemmis, 1986). Many students also perceived the discussion session as providing feedback on their written reflection. One student commented on the pros and cons of journal writing versus group discussion:

'I think it is not necessary to write a journal for every lesson. Group discussion can replace it sometimes. For example, you can finish the lesson and give 10–15 minutes for the small group of 2–3 person to discuss what they have learnt on that day.

I find it troublesome if I do both [journal writing and

discussion]. Because, as I've just said, journal writing can let me have a revision of what have been learnt from the lesson. I think from group discussion I can achieve not only this but also refer to the ideas of other classmates. In case I was sleepy in class or missed some parts of the lecture, group discussion could pave the way for us to stimulate learning mutually among ourselves ... If I have group discussion, the ideas of learned items have been discussed just once. I just write them down once more in my journal. But the real advantage of journal writing is that the lecturer(s) can have a look or check the journal contents. However, the lecturer(s) may not know whether we really understand or can learn from them. Lecturers can see it from the journal writing, but there may be lack of communication among the classmates.'

Students also agreed that group discussion aided learning as can be seen from the following comments:

'It might be a good method to use imagination to solve the problems of clients, because there are many real cases that are unpredictable. It may be because I am a year one student who does not have any idea of this subject. I think that the discussion of the imagined cases can help us to deal with the problem solving. We are not at the level of professional stage. Our thinking is not thoroughly developed. Therefore we can help each other in the discussion of those imagined cases. We discuss which method can help the patients according to the imagined situation. We discuss together to find good methods ... for example, we have different ways of thinking in the discussion.'

Confidence in journal writing

In contrast to the first cycle, students in this cycle rarely mentioned the difficulty of finding an interesting issue to reflect upon, or considered the lack of background knowledge to be a hindrance for reflection. Instead of being more passive in discovering interesting issues, these students were active in using imagined cases in group reflection.

Conclusions for second cycle

The students in the second cycle appeared to have a more positive attitude to and demonstrated greater initiatives towards reflective journal writing. This included a preference for writing reflective journals as opposed to non-reflective ones. The students supported the argument that having strong feelings about a subject makes writing about the subject easier, commenting that if little emotion was engendered in response to an incident, it was less likely to be remembered or to be a subject for reflection.

The use of English as the predominant language in this reflective exercise was a concern and its use should be questioned since it was difficult for (some) students' to express their true feelings in what was not their first language. This area should be explored further.

Within the students' busy schedules, the issue of when to write and how to compose the journal still seemed to be problematic, and so reflective discussion groups were considered as an option to journal writing by some students.

Overall conclusions

Overall, the students were found to have learned about the concept of reflection through engaging in reflective journal writing and by applying their newly acquired academic and practical skills. Though a changed perspective is not expected at this stage of reflective development, students could be seen to be developing the ability to reflect in their daily learning. The implications of this development is that the students may be able to apply these same principles of reflection when they are in clinical practice and dealing with the ill-defined problems of clients and client treatment.

In attempting to illustrate the context of using reflection, we explored the use of reflection through a journal writing process. As we became comfortable with the needs of the students, such as the need for clear instructions and guiding examples, we found that many students were able to use journal writing as a learning tool.

In conclusion, we should state that we had no intention of outlining the limits or the potential of using journal writing as a tool for reflection. Instead, we have attempted to highlight the aspects that we found useful, and, more importantly, to illustrate the context in which it was used. As further exploration is needed to determine the extent of its usefulness for enhancing reflection, we hope the experience presented here will function as a trigger for more research in this area.

Examples from reflective journals of first year students

Student 1

'In this assignment I had to interview someone who had been in hospital. It was the first time I had interviewed a person who I didn't know well (the last time my interviewee was my father). This was a new challenge for me. I found it quite difficult. Also, this interview concerned the personal feelings of my interviewee. I had to consider his feelings and psychological state during the interview. When my interviewee was talking about his deepest feeling related to an unhappy experience, I felt it was quite unnatural and strange for me to write them down formally on paper. This seemed to give him a sense of insecurity and mistrust.

Having completed this assignment, I think that I have several things to improve upon so that I can do the assignment more smoothly next time. First, for the questions I used, I found that questions which included some examples are better and easier for the interviewee to understand. These act as guidelines for the interviewee to answer the questions accurately. If you suddenly ask him some questions which are quite abstract and not easily understandable, the interviewee has no idea how he should answer. Second, I must think carefully about the aim/objective of the assignment before setting out the questions otherwise when you start doing the report, you would find that there is insufficient information. Third, ensure that the interviewee has answered the questions in enough detail. Most important, I need to bear in mind the aim/objective of the assignment when setting the questions for the interview as well as for writing the report.'

Student 2

'I have done the theory assignment. As I have learned from my past mistakes that I made in the interview last time, this time I have done better preparation before having a face-to-face interview with my friend. I have made a list of questions that I would like to ask her during the interview. And I have explained the purpose of the interview to her and the kinds of questions I will ask her.

Although the interviewee is my friend, I still found it difficult when I had to ask about her past experience. As the memories of her mother staying in hospital for a pro-longed period, continuously suffering from cancer pain, suffering from side effects of chemotherapy, having the feeling of helplessness, and then her dying was so painful that she didn't want to talk about it anymore. Therefore I had to pay special attention to her responses and consider her feelings.

In the course of the interview, I had to be aware of her facial expression. Once I found that she seemed to avoid answering my question, I would try to change to another subject and tell her that it is OK if she didn't want to tell me every detail. On the other hand, I gave her sufficient time and patience, so that I could ensure that I wouldn't inter-rupt her expression and also let her know that I was listening very carefully to what she said. Gradually, I found that she was more willing to share her painful experience with me.

I was so glad that she told me at the end of the interview, she was feeling better after she spoke about everything. I felt that I had learned a lot about how to be caring and how to show concern during an interview.'

Chapter 7
Promoting discussion from reflective writing

Kit Sinclair

Introduction

Sharing reflections in group discussion augments the reflective process. Students are able to listen to and reflect upon others' experiences, ask questions and gain different perspectives on their own reflections. By incorporating reflective group discussion into the learning process, students are encouraged to reflect upon learning experiences in class, home reading and relevant work experiences. In an attempt to introduce this approach in an experiential way to clinical educators, reflective journal writing and reflective class discussion became an integral part of a 14-week course on teaching and learning. We found that participants on the course enjoyed this approach and in fact it became central to the participants' learning.

The clinical educators' course entitled *Clinical Education Techniques* followed a set of objectives and assessment. Classes were interactive with participants being expected to take part in discussion, group exercises and role-play. To complete the syllabus, appropriate handouts and teaching materials were provided for each section to be covered.

The participants were asked to keep a reflective journal, to write about a subject of interest from their reading or from their daily work experiences which was relevant to clinical education and the topics we were covering in the syllabus. They were requested to report back to the group at least one item from their reflective journals each week.

The use of the resultant reflective group discussion sessions in class will be described, as well as the reactions of the participants to this learning method – which they found quite new, at first scary, but ultimately quite rewarding.

Journal writing as a precursor to reflective sessions in class

With the help of handouts, the purpose of the course and the use of reflection as a basis for the learning approach was explained. As a precursor to group discussion, participants were asked to keep reflective journals through the week between class sessions. They were given small notebooks to provide some structure to the reflective writing process. In the journals they were asked to record their ideas, feelings and any issues they felt were important in relation to the course on clinical education, their work with students or co-workers during the week, and the reading they did in connection with the course. Reading materials and exercises were provided at the end of each class session to be taken home. They were asked to be prepared to read out and discuss one of these issues at the beginning of class during the following week.

Structure of item disclosure and group process

The participants came to class each week prepared with usually three or four issues for discussion. As the facilitator, I ran the group discussion sessions at the beginning of each class period. The participants were requested to take turns to read out at least one entry from their journal writing.

Although some of the participants were initially unsure and frustrated by a perceived lack of guidelines for the reflective sessions (and for the direction the course should take), they participated regularly in class and had obviously completed the prescribed reading and learning exercises provided for them, and in many cases had reflected on these prior to class.

Class reflection seemed to reinforce their interest. Peer pressure may also have been a factor in their class involvement since they seemed determined to have something to share and discuss in class. They could also see how much reading other members of the class had undertaken by listening in class discussion. The participants were enthusiastic and appeared to be self-motivated in preparing for class and to class discussion. Although they had varying clinical experience, the mutual understanding of the clinical education context and their shared involvement in the healthcare service in Hong Kong stimulated lively discussion. By sharing their thoughts in a small group, they were able to gain further opportunities for their personal reflection on their own disclosures and on issues brought up by other members. By sharing experiences, asking questions, or commenting on each others' reflections, the participants found new areas opening up for consideration which then precipitated further reflection and discussion.

Meeting in the same small group enabled each member to take part in the work of the other members, to support each other, and to respond to the concerns and considerations raised within the group. This mutual support broadened their reflecting and stimulated a degree of risk-taking in personal disclosure. That is, after several sessions, when trust was built up among the members, they appeared more comfortable about sharing more controversial issues. When asked about their motivation to participate in the group discussion, one participant commented:

'I think it was because of the small group arrangement. The atmosphere is built up, and also it is really a responsibility to speak up. If it is your turn and you kept quiet and have nothing to say, then it is quite an embarrassing situation.
... but like in the first lesson, we need you to reinforce (us). But now, we actively bring up issues and participate.'

Another commented:

'I wonder if it is the chair arrangement, where we are debating in a circle, and we can look at each other easily ... and the openness of the participants is very important...
... but I think that the reaction in the group also makes a difference. You feel that it stimulates more discussion ... I think some people maybe want to be part of a very open discussion, but don't know how to start it ... you have to be ready to hear a lot of different views from different students...'

The participants regularly spent one to one-and-a-half hours out of the three-hour evening class in the reflective aspect of the sessions. When asked if they felt we should cut down this part of the programme, they commented that they felt that the reflection was useful and that they looked forward to the ensuing discussions.

Monitoring progress

The journal reading and discussion provided the facilitators with the opportunity to monitor progress on the course and as a measure of where the students were in their understanding of various aspects of the material being covered relevant to clinical education (Wagenaar, 1984). Thus, course materials could be supplemented, discarded or changed as considered necessary. The 'role-play' session, for instance, was chosen on the basis of the background of the participants and their level of interaction at the time. The subsequent discussion of feedback from the role-play brought the participants into further discussion of principles of assessment, which was the next topic in the syllabus.

Resultant raised awareness of reflection and reflective skills

All of the participants were clinical experts in their fields. They knew their respective specialities well. Some of them were new clinical educators. Attending this course made them more aware of the reflective process and its application, and may have increased their conscious reflective activity in their speciality. It appeared to have increased their level of reflection on clinical education and their possible application of reflective techniques with undergraduate students in their clinical settings.

These participants were interested in increasing their clinical teaching skills, so of course much reflection and subsequent discussion which took place during class, referred to the teaching of undergraduate students, student interaction and clinical education feedback. They appear to have gained confidence in their reflective abilities, some commenting on skills they were already using and others commenting on implementation of new ideas gained through their reading and discussion during the course. They also brought up current issues which they needed to problem-solve. In a couple of such instances, a participant would say, '. . . I would like to share with you and hopefully I can find the solution here . . .'

Nystrand & Wiederspiel (1977, cited in Wodlinger, 1990) suggest that students tend to arrive in class with a well-developed set of beliefs and perspectives about teaching and learning in a clinical context usually derived from their own personal experience as students. Participating in the process of exploring one's own and others' experiences and reflections about these experiences allows the students the opportunity to glimpse the world from another's eyes. Participant B confirmed this in her assignment.

'When I stepped into the classroom, I was surprised by the size of the class – only six students – and also the learning style of the class. At first, I was scared about the open discussion as I found it difficult to express my ideas due to the language barrier (needing to use English), and also I was not used to taking the initiative of providing immediate feedback. However, during the open discussion, I picked [up] the other people's ideas that I tried to think of and simultaneously, I appreciated that the handling of interpersonal communication to allow sharing experiences, gave me a sense of contribution.

Although I am glad to experience a high level of acceptance, the fear of exposing my ignorance in front of the teacher and the peers, sometimes really restrained me from participating more actively. However, the reassurance and recognition of my contribution from tutors and the group, were really of great help to solve that problem, by exchanging ideas and feelings with them.'

New perspectives gained through reflection

Throughout the clinical educators' course, the facilitators were involved in responding to ideas which came out of the participants' reflective discussion. They developed a keen sense of the reflective process and became very involved in the reflective reading sessions. It could be seen that they used reflection to focus on specific problems, events or areas of interest which came out of the clinical experience or from their homework reading assignments (Schön, 1983; McCaughtery, 1991; Brookfield, 1993). This reflection could be viewed as purposeful and intentional, self-organised and multifaceted in that they discussed the facts of a situation as well as the attached feelings. (Boud, Keogh & Walker, 1985). These careful examinations of their own experiences and the resultant discussions developed into the formulations of new perspectives and plans for future action. Participant E in her written assignment at the end of the course, commented on her own new perspectives and how she applied them.

'When I started the course "Clinical Education Techniques" in late September last year, I learnt teaching through reflective practice. I was surprised that the technique I was employing was close to the practice. Equipped with the knowledge of the practice learnt from the course, I put new elements into my own reflective sessions with my students. By the end of the placement, we had post-placement conference sessions where all students participated and shared their experiences. It was the time in which I fully used the application of reflection. Students were asked to reflect on their feelings about anything they encountered during the day, besides task-oriented actions. Positive as well as negative experiences were examined. Critical thinking was stressed. Reasons behind an action or feeling were explored, for example, if they felt happy, they were asked to describe the events responsible for the happiness.'

The participants appeared to look forward to the opportunity to share their thoughts and ideas and participated fully in class discussion. Though sometimes they were unable to actually put many thoughts on paper between classes, they had something to share which had been thought through beforehand. Some were more reluctant to speak at first, but gained confidence later. Participant B commented in her assignment:

'I appreciated the exchange of experience in the class discussion as a method of disseminating new information and learning. However, I was dissatisfied with myself (and my own sharing) because I lacked experience in clinical teaching since no student attachment is given to my unit and I believed that learning is established through experience. Such a feeling influenced me for quite a long time. I admitted my 'tunnel vision' eventually and I tried to evaluate my reflective learning ... To a great extent I feel that reflective learning helps me a lot in self-development.'

In another instance the efforts of one participant to brainstorm a concern (the communication barrier between patients and health care professionals) was not written with the view of the journal being read only by herself, but with the view that it would be an issue to be shared and discussed in class, where she could gain opinions from a number of colleagues (Bean & Zulich, 1989).

Participant F commented in his course assignment on the application of reflective learning which he gained during the course with his students in the clinical setting.

'It is interesting that reflection can not only give the above secondary effects [of increased confidence], but also can enhance students' and clinical supervisors' motivation. What is the miracle power behind reflection? With a mind to use reflective tools, it is my usual practice to reply to the students' questions or to clarify their knowledge and concepts in an open way. The words "why", "what", "where", "when", "which" and "how" become the headings of questions. The response seems quite successful. It is not surprising that I am very eager to evaluate my performance with these students as it was the first time that I really acted as a clinical supervisor and interacted with these students for a relatively long period of time. I also had a strong sense of responsibility that I wanted them to be trained as independent therapists, really therapists having the ability to think and to improve by themselves, and to really gain something which is beneficial in their future development. But how? My words can best be summarised by a sentence of the Dean of a well-known School of Management who observed a decade ago that "We need most to teach students how to make decisions under conditions of uncertainty, but this is just what we don't know how to teach." (Pownes, personal communication, 1972, cited in Schön, 1983). Open questioning, high intellectual thinking and correlation are then my strategies after getting to know how to effectively use reflective learning tools.'

My own reflections

I was interested in creating a course which would stimulate experienced clinical educators to be more innovative and alert to the variety of teaching methods which could facilitate students' reflective thinking. I felt that only by experiencing these activities would they become aware of their potential for use with students and be comfortable enough with them to actually implement them in future teaching and learning situations. The evidence from their class discussions, assignments and interviews has shown that involving these clinical educators in the process of using reflective learning in their course has helped them to apply this to work with their students, thus bringing the theory of reflective learning closer to practice for the participants.

Reflective class discussion based on journal writing about clinical and teaching experiences, as well as homework reading, encouraged a thinking focus for group discussion rather than a predominantly task focus like the reporting style usually employed in clinical work. The emphasis on sharing the feeling and emotion as well as the 'doing' aspects of teaching and learning appeared to move the focus to self and self-involvement. It was possible then to draw the participants away from analysing a situation on a technical basis to analysing it on a personal basis, drawing on personal past experience. This may have been possible because these participants had a rich background of experience to draw upon and could discuss their ideas in a small group where, over time, they developed trust in each other and in the facilitators.

I feel that all of those involved in the course, participants and facilitators, have learned to acknowledge and draw more on their own expertise in reviewing and learning about clinical teaching. Reflecting together on the unique or unexpected aspects of a problem or incident facilitated the framing of new questions, the opening of discussion to relevant strategies and objectives to which participants could relate. I found that reflection encouraged the participants to invent novel responses, evaluate their own situation and learn from their and others' experience.

Summary and conclusion

An interactive clinical educators' course was implemented incorporating reflective journal writing and reflective group discussion to develop in clinical educators the ability to use reflection. The ultimate aim of the course was to introduce reflective methods of teaching and learning in clinical education, which could be implemented in clinical education programs for undergraduate students.

The 14-week clinical educators' course entitled *Clinical Education Techniques* followed a clear set of objectives. To cover the syllabus, appropriate handouts and teaching material were provided for each section to be covered and the course employed an interactive and reflective approach. The participants were asked to keep a reflective journal, to write about a subject of interest from their reading or from their daily work experiences which was relevant to clinical education and the topics we were studying in the syllabus. They were requested to report back to the group at least one item from their reflective journals each week. This reflective discussion became the focus of the course.

Reflective group discussion in a small group format was an effective teaching and learning approach. By providing a structure for journal writing and journal disclosure, students could gain confidence in sharing. Journal writing prepared the students for group discussion, equipping them with a focus for reflective sharing. The group rule of one item for disclosure furnished a compromise between the privacy of journal writing and the need for discussion and feedback. The expectation of disclosure allowed them to choose what they wished to discuss, keeping other aspects of their journal writing to themselves.

The structure of journal writing, style of item disclosure, and a sympathetic environment all helped students to overcome the 'scariness' of this new teaching/learning arrangement. Taking part in reflective group discussion with a specific learning focus enabled students to share their own learning, reflect on the observations and learning of others in the group and gain new and different perspectives which might not have been gained through personal reflection alone.

Part III
Synthesising conclusions about curricula

Chapter 8
Encouraging reflective writing

David Kember, Alice Jones, Alice Yuen Loke, Jan McKay,
Kit Sinclair, Harrison Tse, Celia Webb, Frances Kam Yuet Wong,
Marian Wai Lin Wong and Ella Yeung

Introduction

This is the first of the two chapters in which the conclusions
from the five individual or course-based action research
projects are synthesised. The process for this was a comparison between the lessons learnt from the five individual
projects discussed in the chapters in Part II. Regular meetings
of the whole team enabled critical reflection to take place
across projects. Any conclusions drawn from an individual
project could be compared and tested against those from
others.

Essentially this is a process of triangulation (or in this
case 'quintrangulation'?) across courses. The term triangulation has most commonly been used to mean the combination of evaluation or research techniques to study the same
problem, so that a wider and deeper perspective is gained
through the different types of insights resulting from the
methodologies employed (Denzin, 1970). In action research,
Elliott (1991) has used the term in the somewhat different
sense of combining the perspectives and voices of several
sources such as the students, teacher and colleagues. Our
use of the term subsumes both multiple techniques and
multiple voices within each course together with triangulation across projects. The conclusions in this chapter draw
upon at least two of the courses in each case, and often all
five.

The issue dealt with in this chapter is that of how to best
design and implement courses which aim to encourage
reflective writing. Essentially it answers the question of how a
course should be formulated if it is to promote reflection-on-
action and reflective journal writing. The chapter examines
various aspects of courses which appeared to either hinder or

promote student reflection and reflective writing. This was clearly an important aim of the overall project.

In particular, the use of student journals, diaries and regular disclosures was investigated. The problematic issues of assessment and the access of the supervisor to reflections are examined. The study looked at the major blockages to students engaging in reflective writing and sought ways that they could be overcome. Attempts were made to determine which educational factors should be taken into account in the construction of a suitable curriculum and learning environment for reflective writing in professional education courses.

Difficulties of altering previous conceptions of writing

The first conclusion was that students needed an introduction to the concept of reflective writing and on-going help in developing the ability to write reflectively. In the initial cycle of the nursing course, the teachers wished to allow the students to express themselves freely. They expected that students would be able to write in a reflective format with little guidance. This was quickly exposed as a false assumption.

The students found it difficult to break away from previous conceptions of academic writing. Other courses they had taken required them to write in the third person, preferably using a passive tense. Personal observation had been discouraged in favour of citing academic authorities.

Formality is one of the major characteristics of traditional academic writing. Healthcare professionals need a more flexible style of writing because problems in professional practice are sometimes so complicated that there are no formal rules to follow. The quotations below may demonstrate the contradiction of professional practices and traditional writing style.

'In our placement, we have made modification to our knowledge and become more informal. A third person might regard it as doing something wrong, but you have actually used and applied the knowledge in practice without being noticed. If you write this in the journal, others might feel uneasy when they read about the techniques being employed. We have to write formal techniques in our writing. The best thing is to have some background support from academic journals.'

Previous instruction in academic writing had left its mark very effectively. With a few exceptions, the students' initial attempts at reflective writing most closely resembled formal reports. They were replete with evaluations of equipment and facilities and discussion of procedures in hospitals. Criticism focused towards inadequate resource provision. Most of the writing was in the third person and there was little evidence of personal self-reflection.

Many students found initial attempts at reflective writing to be quite a painful experience. The whole concept of reflection was quite alien to many. They had become used to the typical mode of instruction in Hong Kong schools (and one that is common elsewhere as well) in which the teacher delivers a body of content and the students sit passively and try to absorb the material as best they can. Success in this mission is judged by the ability to reproduce selected parts of the body of knowledge in examinations. The majority of the students had become accustomed to thinking of teaching and learning in this way, believing that knowledge was something defined by experts as either right or wrong.

To those with this set of beliefs the concept of reflecting upon their own practice could be quite a rude shock. Instead of course content being selected and delivered by the teacher, the knowledge and experience of the student becomes important. The courses would also have lacked the tight prescriptiveness which would have been a feature of most of the students' previous education.

> '... at the beginning, I really had to think very hard, picking issues to talk of or to enter as a reflective journal. But towards the end of the module, I found it more spontaneous and easier to link up the experience to my learning ... not only in understanding, but as I have said, you will spontaneously pick up reflective learning yourself.'

The majority adjusted to a more student-centred style of teaching and learning and eventually came to prefer it. However, at the outset these new learning experiences could be both difficult and unpleasant. The affective dimension to coming to grips with reflective writing is dealt with in detail in Chapter 10.

We came to see reflective writing as an ability which took time to develop and, for some, was quite difficult to achieve. Formal education normally requires a style of writing which is virtually the antithesis of reflective writing. Many students find it hard to unlearn their conception of impersonal academic writing and to record their personal reflections. In our courses, however, we demonstrated the students' capability of achieving this through careful instructional planning and frequent feedback.

Journal writing, therefore, needs to be treated as an ability to be developed over time. Courses must allow space and time for this development to take place. There needs to be provision for frequent feedback on what is written. In providing feedback lecturers/tutors, clinical supervisors and fellow students have a role to play.

Introducing the concept of reflection

To develop the students' ability to write reflectively it was necessary to have both introductory sessions and reinforcement throughout the course. The on-going development mainly came through periodic feedback on submitted journals.

The nursing course had an initial workshop which served as a formative model for introducing students to the concept of reflection. The concept was introduced to the students using the illustration of a model of reflection (Boud, Keogh & Walker, 1985). Some of the students' reflective journals from the first cycle were given as examples to demonstrate the progress of reflection progression. The nursing course aimed to facilitate students' reflection upon contemporary nursing issues. Students were encouraged to write down their thoughts or impressions concerning the identified issues provided by lecturers as their reflection exercises. Feedback was given to the students each time they completed one of the four required journal submissions as guidance for the future reflective process.

The occupational therapy course had a similar introductory session during one of their first tutorials. Students were introduced to the concepts of reflective learning and given explanatory handouts. They were required to reflect, analyse and critically evaluate activities they undertook during the class in relation to their past experience, observations, and feelings. Discussion was engendered on the concepts of reflection and its application in learning. Reflective journal writing was introduced and guidelines for writing journals distributed. Students were asked to keep a journal of personal feelings and reactions to some learning activities and then focus on an issue that they felt was of particular significance.

About half way through the semester, a tutorial session was spent discussing 'reflective learning' and the problems encountered in attempting to write their journals. Interviews conducted at the end of the course showed that students had generally evolved a working definition of a reflective journal as one which showed personal feelings, ideas or impressions, and would help to identify problems in their learning. However, a non-reflective journal just showed the processes of the clinical events with students soon forgetting what was written in this type of journal.

Students in all the courses seemed to appreciate being provided with good examples of reflective writing from previous students. When providing examples it was found to be better to offer several with as much variety of good practice as possible. There was a tendency for students to model their writing on the examples, so if a limited number of samples were provided, the format of writing could be constrained to one similar to the models on offer.

Format for reflective writing

The format for reflective writing and the periodicity of requiring students to complete journal entries was a function of the course. Clinical educators were provided with a small notebook for journal entries. The intention of using notebooks was to avoid formal academic report-like writing and to encourage the journals to be used more like personal diaries. Provision of notebooks helped to demonstrate that journal writing was different from other forms of academic writing which are word-processed and handed in on standardised sheets of paper. The students were encouraged to make notes on readings and reflect at home, at work and during classes. It was reasonable not to restrict the structure of the journal while students' intrinsic interest was being encouraged.

The other courses had more structured arrangements as a result of the differing focuses for reflection. Typically students were asked to hand in journal entries at intervals during the course. These were not assessed but feedback on the reflective writing was provided. At the end of the course students were required to write a longer piece of reflective writing which drew upon the earlier work. This final piece of writing was part of the assessment so that reflective writing was seen as integral to the course and students were motivated to take it seriously.

In the radiography course the reflective process was initially encouraged as an exercise separate from the clinical assignments that were already in place. The students were asked to keep journal notes on each placement they attended. They were asked to review the placement in terms of the objectives to be achieved, and to analyse their own success in achieving them.

After two cycles of clinical experience with students writing separate reflective analyses, it was felt that the separation of the reflective exercise from the more formal clinical assignments reduced the students' concentration on the reflection exercise. Rather than make the reflection exercise additional to the clinical assignments, it was agreed to reformulate the assignments to more clearly include the reflective process. At the first level, for example, the assignments now require the students to discuss their own ability to perform and assess the outcomes for the examinations and procedures they are analysing. Similar adjustments have been made at the second and third levels of clinical experience.

The physiotherapy course was interesting in that it had a quite different format for reflection from the journal writing used by the other courses in the form of a learning contract. This has been discussed in detail in Chapter 5.

Structure of journals

No structure for the journals was provided in two of the courses, one being nursing. Students were free to express their views however they wished. Their discussion could be based on library sources and references. However, it was emphasised that their interpretations of the ideas and the integration of nursing practice were of ultimate importance. The clinical educators were asked simply to write something in their journal in preparation for each of the weekly classes.

Occupational therapy journals were semi-structured. Brief guidelines about journal writings were provided to occupational therapy students although they were not asked to follow them strictly. Students were recommended to start with describing their experience of learning during a particular learning activity, such as an interview situation or visits. Then they could focus on some aspects that impressed them most and explain their feelings in relation to their strengths, capacities, fears, weaknesses, biases, etc.

An early attempt at structuring journals in the radiography course showed that the provided structure should be kept to a minimum. Students were initially given a list of objectives for each placement and asked to reflect on their progress towards achieving them during the clinical period. Rather than stimulating reflection, the provision of objectives reduced most of the students to ticking objectives met and making brief comments on others.

The revised reflective journal for the radiography students was divided into sections. Firstly students were asked to review their previous experience in relation to the clinical objectives, then to state what progress they would like to achieve over the course of the clinical block. They then set specific objectives and reviewed progress for each individual placement, and finally made an assessment of overall progress at the completion of the block.

The students were also expected to complete written exercises during the periods of clinical experience that were designed to encourage them to investigate and reflect upon clinical settings against their theoretical background. The level of reflection was expected to increase as the course progressed. At the first stage they were required to note and discuss the manner and degree to which certain examination types were used in a particular clinical setting. The second stage required them to produce case studies of examinations from a series of placements offering different experience. The students reported on cases that differed, for some reason, from the normal department procedure. At the third stage the students made a comprehensive analysis of two clinical settings they attended which included an analysis of their own strengths and weaknesses as a member of the team. At each stage the clinical assignments were incorporated into tutorial classes at the completion of the clinical period.

The experience in the radiography course of providing students with an over-structured journal format suggests that the provision of extensive structuring in journals is likely to stifle individual reflection and lead to stereotyped responses. However, the provision of one or two headings, in courses which desired students to reflect on specified topics, did seem to serve a useful purpose. For the two courses which were more open about the topic of reflection, an unstructured format seemed essential.

Assessment of journal writing

The issue of assessment for grading purposes poses a dichotomy for courses intending to incorporate journal writing. Assessing journal entries can discourage the process of private reflection. There is also the obvious problem of what might have been written for the student alone becoming transformed into something quite different in an attempt to gain better marks. Assessing journal entries tends to discourage criticism and leads to polishing of work and a more academic style rather than spontaneous reflection. However, if the written entries are not assessed, students tend to take journal writing less seriously or even not do it at all. Students are highly assessment-driven and course-marking schemes are usually treated as guidelines for the relative importance of components of courses. This dilemma between discouraging free expression and not motivating students to take the journal writing seriously was illustrated by student quotations in Chapter 4.

If the type of journal writing is loosely structured, the importance of examining journal entries and providing feedback is particularly high. Without any feedback there is no mechanism for improving the reflective writing. For example, a radiography student stressed the motivational effect of feedback when he talked about assessment of journals. The importance of the writing making a significant contribution to the assessment is also apparent.

'If marks are given, it gives some sort of motivation to do it. The motivational effect, however, is not great. For example, if it carries five marks, I would be willing to hand it in. If I hand it in, at least I might have three marks. The most serious problem is having no feedback. They have to show respect for the work of other people. They need to go through, correct and talk with us when it is given back to us. This would be the most important question. For instance, even if they tell me I get full marks, I won't care much as I don't know where my paper is right now and they won't give it back to you.'

Compromise position

In the main our courses strove for a middle position which retained an element of freedom and privacy in journal writing while integrating it within the course and incorporating elements from the journal writing in the assessment. It was recognised that at least some early journal writing needed to be examined so that developmental feedback could be given. Grading this early writing, though, did not seem conducive to encouraging freedom of expression. The problem of students failing to take reflective writing seriously if it was not assessed was dealt with by including a final piece of reflective writing in the assessment. This usually drew upon earlier writing in some way so that those were taken seriously also. For example, in the nursing course the students were required to submit four journals at regular intervals throughout the course and a final reflective paper. The journals were unstructured and not marked. They were handed in so that feedback could be given to students as guidelines for their future reflective activities. A final reflective paper, which was assessed, was to be submitted after the experience of all the dialogue sessions. It was intended that the final paper should be distilled from the four journals previously submitted. Students themselves regarded marking as an effective and essential feedback to their assignments. In an interview at the end of the course, one of the students in the nursing course stated:

'In fact marking is a good thing. Without it, I would not be able to know the quality of my journals. After they had read our journals, they told us whether the content was relevant to the topic during group discussion. But I think it was not enough for every one of us. I would be able to know my performance better if the papers are marked.'

An argument for having at least some reflective writing assessed comes from the course which had the greatest difficulty in persuading students to participate in journal writing. Journal writing was introduced in the physiotherapy course as a voluntary element but the majority of students felt they had enough to cope with without having to keep a journal as well! However, a handful were agreeable to trying it out. The plan for keeping reflective diaries on an on-going basis during the clinical placement raised little interest not only among students but, as was found out later, also with staff. However, despite that, most of the students tended to agree that reflection would assist with better understanding of, for example, a problem or interaction and hence, could pave the way for improvement. The main reason given for the students (and some clinical educators) being unwilling to write journals on an on-going basis was because it would consume too much of their time which they desperately needed for searching for relevant medical and other information necessary for the appropriate treatment of their patients. Whether they were able to do this or not would affect their chances of passing the placement.

The conclusion reached was that courses needed to adapt their format so that students perceived reflective writing as an intrinsic component. However, the process of adapting the course format needed both sensitivity and experimentation. The course elements which signify centrality are assessing journals, examining the writing in them and requiring students to disclose at least some journal entries in tutorial discussion. Yet if handled insensitively, each of these measures could inhibit private journal writing. The courses in this study attempted to evolve a format which signified the importance of journal writing while still retaining some element of the sanctity of personal reflections.

There is no easy answer to this dichotomy. The courses studied for this project provided examples of the influence of assessing or not assessing journal entries. Some intermediate positions were also evolved in which the bulk of the journal entries remained private but work derived from them was assessed so that students had some incentive to participate in journal writing. In deciding if assessing reflective writings is appropriate or not, one should consider the format and the nature of the writings.

Frequency with which journal entries are examined

A further aspect of the dichotomy over the privacy of journal writing is whether, and if so, how often the lecturer reads what is written in the journal. The issue of the frequency with which journal entries are examined is bound up with the purpose for which they are examined. The courses in this study formed a spectrum in terms of how often the lecturers examined the students' journals. For the clinical educators' course the journals formed the basis of weekly discussion and of a final assignment but were not required to be handed in.

For the first round of the occupational therapy course, students discussed their journal entries in formal discussion sessions in class about half-way through the course. In an interview at the end of the course, students generally showed the need for more discussions about the content of their journal. The quotations below are examples of some of their statements.

- 'Maybe the lecturer can arrange more discussions on the journal writing. Discussions can help students to know what they have learnt in the visit or in the journal writing. The lecturer can further elaborate our information.'

- 'Ideally, the discussion should be before and after the journal writing, but I know that there is not enough time for discussion. So, I think the discussion should take place after journal writing.'

As a result of this feedback, arrangements were devised in all of the courses for earlier and more frequent disclosure or examination of journal writing. The disclosure could be in the form of handing in journal entries to the lecturer for comment and feedback. Alternatively, or as well as, part of the journal entries could form the basis for small group discussion sessions. Either approach allowed the students to gain feedback on their reflective writing and provided them with encouragement to engage in further writing.

The arrangements indicate that various compromise positions were adopted. Excessive intrusion into journals would inhibit personal reflection and change the writing to a more publicly 'acceptable' form. Yet no examination means that the lecturers gain no feedback on understanding of the course material and no opportunity to monitor and shape the students' development as reflective writers.

Overall the conclusion was that examination of journal entries needed to be reasonably frequent if students were new to reflective writing. Without frequent disclosure there was no opportunity to provide feedback on the students' development as reflective writers and no chance to assist the students to evolve away from ingrained conceptions of academic writing towards a more open reflective style. The type of feedback can be varied and may include written feedback and tutorial discussions.

Conclusion

This chapter has discussed a range of elements within the teaching and learning environment. In each it has shown how the context impinges upon reflective learning. The chapter has provided some suggestions about which factors are important and discussed how they might be configured.

There are few aspects of teaching which have a clear uni-directional impact on reflective writing; rather a course often has to evolve towards an intelligent position between dichotomies. The curriculum and teaching format needs to achieve a balance between factors which act in combination and are to some extent sensitive to each other.

Courses can differ markedly in terms of their content, the

background of the students, the institutional climate and the time and resources available. Each of these contextual elements should be taken into account in configuring a curriculum to promote reflective writing. Curriculum planning should draw upon established wisdom but interpreted in a way which is sensitive to the context.

Action research approach

Putting such a curriculum into practice in a situation will undoubtedly require further fine-tuning to achieve a balanced arrangement which suits a particular course and learning environment. There are suggestions in this chapter which should help the initial curriculum design. The action research approach described is also appropriate for dealing with implementation and adaptation to a particular context.

An important element of the approach has been its participative and collaborative nature. An aspect of this which has perhaps been understated so far in the chapter has been the involvement of the students. The writing has focused at the meta-project level where findings were synthesised from five course-level action research projects. Student involvement has been much more apparent at the course level, where they have been contributors to each of the individual course projects. Indeed it has been essential to have the involvement of, and input from, the many students enrolled on these courses. Students' reflection on the course experience has directly or indirectly influenced all of the strategies described. An example of the value of this input is given by the following suggestions on how to introduce the concept of reflection which will be incorporated into future cycles.

- 'I think if the lecturer lets the students in year 2 or year 3 or some graduate students to tell the year 1 students what is the importance or the significance of reflective journal writing. I think it will be more exciting than an introduction by the lecturer ... It may arouse their interest and they will become more active...'

- 'I think that the lecturer has to explain the main aim of reflective journals at the beginning of the year. And the lecturer may use some guidelines for the student and use journals of the past students as examples. And the lecturer may help the students to discuss some topics related to the lecture in class. Then, after discussion, we can jot down some notes and write the reflective journal for the lecturer. I think this is the best way.'

To receive this type of response it is important to have a good relationship with students so that informal feedback on teaching can be gathered. It is also important to have a rigorous evaluation of the courses which is sensitive to student opinion. In this study most of the data were qualitative and gained from interviews. Data were also gathered from student journals. These were examined to determine the level of reflectivity reached by students, and seeing whether the courses were meeting their objectives (Kember, Jones, Loke, McKay, Sinclair, Tse, Webb, Wong, Wong & Yeung, 1999).

At the meta-project level, the collaborative and inter-departmental nature of the project has been important. Collaboration complicated the logistics of the project, as even arranging a meeting time when all were free was quite difficult. However, the logistical difficulties were outweighed by the benefits from the cross-fertilisation of ideas and experiences between courses and teachers.

Chapter 9
Facilitating critical discussion

David Kember, Alice Jones, Alice Yuen Loke, Jan McKay,
Kit Sinclair, Harrison Tse, Celia Webb, Frances Kam Yuet Wong,
Marian Wai Lin Wong and Ella Yeung

Introduction

This is the second of the two chapters in which conclusions
about course and curriculum design are synthesised. This
chapter examines the way in which reflective journal writing
can be used as a stimulus for critical reflection through group
discussion. Many courses encourage or require students to
individually reflect upon their practice, usually through the
writing of a journal. Of these courses, a significant proportion has a further stage in which students share some element
of their written reflection with fellow students and/or tutors.
This discussion normally takes place in a tutorial or seminar,
with the journal entries serving as a starting point or focus for
the discussion.

The chapter examines the impact of the following contextual elements on class discussions based upon written
reflection:

- the relationship between journal writing and tutorial
  discussion
- the dichotomy of making private written reflections
  public through tutorial discussions
- group size
- the physical arrangement for discussions in class
- inter-group interaction
- the relationship between and the interaction of educators
  and learners
- tape recording of discussion sessions

The synthesised conclusions considered how these various
aspects of the courses appeared to either hinder or promote
student reflection and discussion of that reflection.

Comparison was made between two or more of the courses studied in each case. For many of the conclusions all five courses were drawn upon.

Journal writing by itself is seen as a valuable stimulus to encourage reflection upon practice (e.g. Wagenaar, 1984; Hahnemann, 1986; Bean & Zulich 1989; Cameron & Mitchell, 1993). Discussion of reflective writing can add further dimensions to the experience. Firstly the students share ideas – they benefit from the insights of their fellow students as well as their own. Many of the students also perceive the discussion sessions as providing feedback upon their written reflection. Finally, if the tutorial gels, the critical discourse will serve to develop collective understanding.

The strategy of basing tutorial discussion upon reflective writing can be located within a wider spectrum of interest and research on tutorial discussion and small-group teaching in general. Within this wider context there has been research into relevant aspects of group behaviour, such as group size, group dynamics, social pressure, group decisions, leadership nature, group structure and their inter-relationships (see Zander, 1979; Jaques, 1991, ch. 2, for reviews). There are also several books which give valuable advice on how to conduct small group teaching (e.g. Habeshaw, Habeshaw and Gibbs, 1984; Jaques, 1991).

Despite this body of expertise there are still probably any number of tutors who face such perennial problems as unprepared groups, discussions dominated by individuals and those awful silences. There are even greater numbers of students with complaints about boring, irrelevant or unproductive tutorials. This chapter does not guarantee to eliminate boring tutorials. It does though, provide insights into how journal writing can prepare students for tutorial or group discussion and help in promoting valuable critical discussion. For this wider issue of how to conduct stimulating and relevant small-group teaching the conclusions presented in this chapter do have relevance. Basing the discussion on journal writing usually resulted in students being prepared for the tutorials and often generated lively discussion and debate.

Relationship between journals and tutorial discussion

Journal writing can be a useful exercise in itself. Within a taught course it is also commonly a precursor to critical discussion within tutorial groups. The content and quality of journal writing can influence the nature and substance of the dialogue. This in turn contributes to or, in some cases largely constitutes the content and effectiveness of the course.

This section examines the way journal writing was utilised within discussion or tutorial sessions. For the nursing and clinical educators' courses, journal writing formed the initial substance or starting point for discussion topics. The other three courses used the journal writings more as a way of revisiting recent clinical experience sessions and collectively reflecting upon them.

For the clinical educators, reading of journal items formed a major component of the weekly class discussion. Each class member was expected to read out at least one item from his or her journal. They found discussion of journal entries useful as it could result in more profound insights into the topic. As one student reported:

'Take for example the discussion on the difference between deep and superficial learning. Actually, I hadn't thought about it before. But during the sharing of the reflective journal, someone had a little discussion on this. Suddenly, I just realised that, take for example myself, during my undergraduate study, I really learned in a very superficial way. And also, I linked it to some experience when I'm teaching students.'

Tutorial discussion in the radiography group was developed from experiences recorded by the students in their journals. Each student was asked to contribute one item they had noted for discussion within the group. The discussions were very free-ranging. Not every student necessarily contributed an item though they were all encouraged to express opinions.

There was evidence that the combination of journal writing and discussion resulted in more effective learning outcomes than if the two elements were discrete. The quotation below was made by a radiography student on the basis of his three year's experience in the course.

'If we can't think of anything at that moment, that is the things which are not written down, we can find it out during the discussion. At the same time, knowledge will be greater as we may think of something suddenly which we had not thought of before. Thus, I think if two of them are combined, I think it will be better. It may not be so effective if they are separated.'

Discussion drew out more from the journal entries both to the writer and to others in the tutorial group. It was also observed that the outcomes of the discussion contributed to successive journal entries.

The combination of journal writing with group discussion helped to avoid some of the most common problems of tutorials or seminars. The process of writing served as preparation for the meeting. Not every student was prepared for every discussion, but the level of preparation was higher than that usually found in tutorials, where it is by no means uncommon to find that no students have made any preparations, or perhaps just the student selected to write a seminar paper for the particular session. The preparatory aspect of journal writing also helps in overcoming the common problem of the deadly silence in tutorials. If students know they will have to contribute at least one item from their journals to the discussion, there is at least a starting point for a discussion.

Making reflections public

There is something of a dichotomy in moving from journal writing to tutorial discussion if the journals are seen as a private domain for personal feelings. Students may feel constrained from free introspection on their impressions and feelings if they know that their journal writings will be made public. Yet without some element of disclosure there can be no discussion and no opportunity for sharpening insights through communal critical reflection. The way this issue was dealt with was to establish ground rules at the outset of the course. In some cases these were proposed by the teacher and accepted by the class. In other cases the ground rules were developed in more tacit ways as a kind of group norm.

The ground rule in the clinical educators' course was that students should read out and comment on at least one entry from their journals during the weekly classes. Students could, therefore, choose to keep some reflections private while still making a contribution to the class discussion. In practice the possibility of keeping reflections private was rarely used, as students tended to read all their reflections. Possibly the small size of the class and the coherence it developed dissipated any desire to keep reflections private.

The nursing course was one with less formally established ground rules. The class was divided into eight groups of eight to ten students for small group dialogue. Some students at first were quiet in some of the groups. The problem was overcome very quickly when it seemed to be a norm that everyone in the group had to speak before the session ended. There was variation between groups with each group establishing its own ground rules and peer pressure ensuring that all made some contribution.

Overall, it turned out that we may have been more sensitive about the issue of disclosing reflective writing than we need have been. Keeping reflections private did not seem to be a strong issue with the students. There seemed to be a recognition of the benefits of sharing reflections. They generally recognised that making reflections public not only benefited other participants in the group but also benefited the speaker. This is illustrated by the retrospection of one student.

'... I used to share what I reflected with somebody. It doesn't matter who, maybe you, maybe my students, or maybe my husband or maybe a friend. Discussion strengthens my points and thinking, and because I know that it is my weakness to find a way to express it. In that reflection, I reflect on that too. So, it will lead me to a way of solving it.'

Group size and arrangement for discussions

The courses had a range of group size and differing arrangements for holding the discussion sessions. The size of the groups were more a function of available resources than conscious curriculum planning, though the variation between courses did permit an examination of the influence of group size on reflective discussion.

The clinical educators' course had an unusually generous staff to student ratio, because the course was new and lecturers volunteered to participate. When classes were held, the six students and three facilitators were involved in most journal reading sessions. The classroom was arranged so that chairs were in a circle and discussion could flow easily among all participants. Students were well satisfied with the group size which encouraged the interactions of participants.

The radiography group was divided into six tutorial groups, with the number per group ranging between nine and eleven participants, excluding the facilitator. The discussions sessions occurred in the week following the end of the clinical placement period and were incorporated into regular tutorial

groups. When students were asked about the optimal discussion group size, their preference ranged from between six
and ten participants. The statements below give some reasons
for the proposed arrangement from a student's point of view.

'I think around five to six people, but it should not exceed
ten people. If it is over ten there is someone who is shy and
may not be able to speak out ... otherwise, there will be
someone who will not say anything. They won't speak out
even if they think of something.'

The nursing course had to adopt more formal arrangements as it had a staff to student ratio of three lecturers to run
the course for a class of 80. The class was divided into eight
groups with approximately ten students in each group. Two
of the lecturers had to work with three groups in one session,
and the other one was responsible for two groups. Students
were asked to take turns to chair their groups, with some
groups functioning better than others in this arrangement.
The following are the opinions of two students about the
arrangement.

- 'I have mentioned that we often had group discussion
  without a tutor beside us. I think a tutor should stay
  with us during the discussion. Maybe our tutor had no
  time to do so.'

- 'You mean there are differences between group discussion with and without tutors present?' (researcher)

- 'It is better if a tutor gives us stimulation at the right
  time during discussion.'

- 'The number of lecturers is limited. Furthermore, they
  have their own restrictions. For example, Tutor A was
  responsible for three groups. It was difficult for her to
  take care of each student's need. They could not spend
  too much time with each group, so they could only get a
  very superficial understanding of each group's discussion and they could not notice the direction of our
  discussion. As a result, the guidance they were able to
  give us was limited.'

The experiences of the different courses show that group
size is important – if the group is too large reflective discussion will be inhibited. The conclusions we drew are in line
with research into how the characteristics of groups alter
with size (Rice, 1971; Jaques, 1991). Groups with fewer than

six members need little structure or leadership and tend to be very fluid; more than six members and individuals become less constrained by the norms of the group and more formal structuring and leadership emerges if the group is to be successful. Group sizes above about 12 are unsuitable for reflective discussion as full face-to-face interaction decreases and sub-groups begin to appear. If resources only allow for class sizes above 12, it is better to split the class into smaller groups – if necessary without a tutor as a leader. The arrangement adopted in the nursing course of a lecturer moving between two or three groups is not ideal but is better than attempting to generate reflective discussion in large groups.

When the class is large, a pyramid strategy can be used. At the initial stages discussion can take place between pairs of students. This ensures that everyone can contribute and develop a position on the selected topic. The discussion from the pairs is then taken to somewhat larger focus groups. In a large class with one teacher, these will have to be student-led but the teacher can move between the groups. The final stage is at the whole class level when a spokesperson from each focus group reports the group conclusion. There can be a wider discussion at this level but it obviously becomes difficult for everyone to have a direct voice as the class becomes larger. However, the pyramid structure means that everyone can have input and a voice, even if this may be passed on indirectly in the latter stages of the exercise.

Inter-group interaction

The extent of collaborative reflection is also an important issue. Deliberate arrangements were made to increase the extent of collaborative reflection in the nursing course, from small group discussions to inter-group discussions. These inter-group dialogue sessions aimed to provide opportunities to share ideas as some of the groups had become rather restricted in the breadth of their discussions. In the inter-group sessions fellow students were invited to challenge conceptual schemes presented. It was hoped that this would broaden horizons or bring forward new perspectives for the subsequent dialogue and journal writing.

In order to broaden the perspectives of students and induce further stimulation, a combined group discussion, which we called *inter-group* dialogue was planned. The large class was originally divided into eight small groups, each concentrating on one theme in their reflective learning. In this instance the eight groups were brought altogether in a large class setting. Each group would have 15 minutes to present their learning and insights about the particular theme that they were dealing with. They had the freedom to choose the method of presentation, or the number of group members involved. The common practice usually involved a few members speaking on behalf of the group but all group members would present themselves on the stage to respond to questions and comments in the 15 minutes after presentation. After the group had the opportunity to express their ideas and reflections to the class, the class would then engage in dialogue with the group, raise questions, challenge their viewpoints, or share similar experience.

This arrangement was found to have at least two effects. One was that the group itself had an opportunity to review and revisit what it had learnt in the process. This organisation of ideas by itself could be reflective, mapping out the analysis of the issue at hand. Secondly, the large class could take an 'outsider' view, as well as an empathetic view of the issue. As 'outsiders' of the group, they could highlight viewpoints which were different from the orientation taken by the small group. However, very often members in the large class also could converge their experience with that of the small group. The former situation could serve the purpose of challenging assumptions, and the latter, confirming hypotheses. These two components were essential to higher levels of reflection.

Students also found the two types of discussion groups useful and their functions different. The comment below was made by a nursing student when being asked about the impact of small group discussion.

'In different groups, our discussion was different. As our experiences are not the same, everybody is likely to express their own ideas ... some classmates show their anger from their work, we then have better advice to give to each other. This can allow us to have a better discussion and let us learn more.'

The inter-group sessions did seem to bring forward new perspectives.

'We can concentrate on subject matter in intra-group discussion. The ideas may not be creative enough. However in inter-group discussion, our ideas can stimulate the others to think from other points of view. That is why we have more new ideas in inter-group discussion. It helps us to think deeply.'

Tape recording

Tape recordings of class discussions were originally introduced purely as an observation or research technique. However, in the clinical educators' course, taping quickly assumed a function which had never been envisaged at the outset. The students saw the tapes as a valuable learning resource and requested individual copies. All journal disclosures and discussion sessions were recorded. The recordings eventually achieved such perceived importance that concern was expressed if recording was halted for reasons such as the tape running out. The conversation would be halted until the tape was replaced in case valuable discussion was omitted from the tape.

The students seemed to view the recordings of their discussions as a substitute for lecture notes. There was little in the way of content delivery in the class sessions. There were set readings but the students soon came to see that the essential 'content' of the course was the collective critical reflections of the class discussion. They, therefore, wanted a full record of this discussion. Tape recording gave them a full and accurate record without restricting their participation, which note-taking might have done. The content of the tape recording could be used as a metaphorical stimulation for reflection and play a significant role in enhancing a breakthrough from routine, as one of the students stated in the tutorial session.

'These two days, I thought about teaching methodology. At first I couldn't reflect. Then I listened to the recording again and again. I quite agree that most of the students [the receivers] need to have extrinsic and intrinsic factors...'

Other courses either decided to do no recording at all, or made occasional recordings of selected discussion sessions for evaluation purposes. The rationale for not recording sessions was that discussion could be inhibited or that having a record of the discussion served no useful purpose. There was some evidence of the inhibiting effect of the presence of tape recorders in the nursing course. In the initial stages of the course taping of some sessions was attempted with unsuitable insensitive tape recorders. To obtain an audible recording students had to hand round the recorder. When suitable equipment was used, however, students usually forgot about its presence after a while.

Given the value accorded the tapes by the clinical education students, it seems worthwhile to ask students whether they would find tape recordings of their discussion sessions useful and if so whether all consent to the taping of sessions. No recording should be attempted, though, unless suitable unobtrusive equipment is available. The lecturers found taping class sessions useful. The tapes provided a valuable stimulus for their reflections on their teaching and a valuable component of evaluations of the courses.

Conclusion

The chapter has examined critical discussion based upon reflective writing. One conclusion is that the writing process can serve as very good preparation for a tutorial discussion. Indeed, given the levels of discussion within each of the five courses, it can be seen as a very good strategy for avoiding the perennial problems of students coming to tutorials and seminars with limited preparation so that there is little or no discussion.

The benefits, though, go well beyond ensuring that discussion takes place. Students found that the combination of journal writing and critical discussion with colleagues led to insights and knowledge which would not have come from either element alone. Reflective journals in combination with peer discussion proved to be a potent force towards students constructing their own understanding. A range of elements within the teaching and learning environment have been discussed, in each case attempting to show how the variables impinge upon reflective learning. There are few aspects of teaching which have a clear unidirectional impact on reflective thinking. Rather a course often has to evolve towards an intelligent position. The curriculum and teaching format needs to achieve a balance between factors which act in combination and are to some extent sensitive to each other.

This chapter has provided some suggestions about which factors are important and how they might be configured. Putting them into practice in a particular course or situation will undoubtedly require further fine-tuning or action research to achieve a balanced arrangement which suits a particular course and learning environment.

Part IV
The nature of reflection

Chapter 10
The affective dimension of reflection

Marian Wai Lin Wong, David Kember, Frances Kam Yuet Wong
and Alice Yuen Loke

Introduction

This is the first of two chapters in which we re-examine the
nature of reflection. We analyse data from the extensive collection of journal entries and interviews needed for the evaluations and investigations carried out for the work described
in the previous chapters. In most cases the analysis is from the
new perspective of looking at the nature of reflection, rather
than issues concerning teaching approaches or curriculum
design. We also draw upon are the conclusions developed in
earlier chapters about course design and teaching methods
appropriate for developing reflective thinking.

This chapter deals with affective aspects of reflection. It
was the purpose of this part of the overall project to investigate the students' affective responses during reflective
learning, and to explore the consequences for personal and
professional development. The analysis on which it is based
examined students' affective statements about reflective
thinking. Initial statements often showed negative reactions.
By the end of the course, though, most students made more
positive affective statements about reflective thinking. Having a supportive environment provided by faculty and fellow
students seemed important when making this transition. The
nature of this support is not included in Figure 10.1 showing
our analysis of affective feelings on reflection, but there is a
section towards the end of the chapter which reports our
insights into how students can be eased through the initial
painful encounters with reflective thinking towards more
productive and comfortable positions.

Awareness of the affective responses and understanding of
the affective functioning that was provoked in returning to

experience appears to affect the reflection process. Boud, Cohen & Walker (1993) identified 'barriers' to reflective learning which concern emotional factors and may inhibit learners entering into a new experience. They also showed though, that emotions sometimes serve as a shield to the stress of returning to past experience. However, these may spawn affective consequences that make reflection impossible. If students and practitioners are to learn how to reflect upon their daily experience, they need to know more about the nature of the affect and its impact on reflective learning. They need to envision the consequences of reflection and recognise the implications of the emotional presence during the process.

There is a lack of research and examination of the role of affective responses in reflective practice and its impacts on those who are learning to reflect upon the phenomenon of practice. In this chapter though we show that affective responses to attempts to create the type of curriculum elements intended to develop reflective practitioners were a paramount concern of the students. How well the students coped with this type of teaching and learning had a crucial impact upon whether critical reflection occurred.

Analysis

The conclusions presented in this chapter were drawn from the journal and essay entries and in-depth unstructured interviews with students in the nursing course. Only six sets of complete data were used for analysis. The characteristics of the learners' affective status were recognised by a content analysis of these data. The interactions of the learners in dialogue sessions were observed and recorded. The data from the observation contributed to the construction of questions for the subsequent interviews.

On the whole, most of their feelings were identified from the data obtained from interviews. There were students handicapped by devastating feelings while others were able to engage actively in the reflection process by the acknowledgement of these mixed emotions. Only a few managed to describe their feelings when they were reflecting in their journals at the interface of the individual role and their practice. Others did not demonstrate awareness of their feelings upon reflection, or they chose not to express their feelings. The denial of the affective responses did not appear to help them to enter into any reflection. The source of these personal feelings should be confronted and transformed with the standard of rationality according to Boud, Cohen & Walker (1993).

By the final stage of analysis it had become apparent that a number of the identified themes were related. The most apt way of representing these relationships seemed to be a hierarchical clustering. The feelings could be readily sub-divided into positive and negative. Under both positive and negative divisions there were two further layers of categories.

Figure 10.1 shows the hierarchical categorisation of the themes which were identified. There are three levels of categorisation. Firstly affective responses were divided into negative or uncomfortable responses, and more positive feelings displaying an increased comfort level. Secondly, the identified themes were grouped into clusters. The left-hand side of the table gives the two main themes. In the remainder of the chapter the themes within their clusters are amplified and illustrated with typical quotations from the examined transcripts.

It should be stressed at this point that the categories apply to affective responses. They cannot be used to 'label' students since individuals could and did make affective statements which were both positive and negative. Indeed a major aspect of the findings discussed below, was a common shift from negative expressions about reflection to more positive ones.

Uncomfortable feelings

The initial level of analysis divided the expressed feelings into positive and negative categories. The stimulating and challenging feelings of their learning experience were frequently reported as the positive aspects of the students' affective reactions. Concerning the negative reflective experience, anxiety, fear and discontent were the three predominant threats expressed. The negative feelings are dealt with first here first because they reflect the temporal ordering of emotions expressed by quite a number of students. Within the initial division we will work down and across the hierarchy, examining the three main sub-divisions:

- fear of new learning methods in general
- fear of specific aspects of a new learning method
- workload

Each of these sub-divisions had a number of themes clustered within them. The themes are illustrated with quotations from journals and interview transcripts.

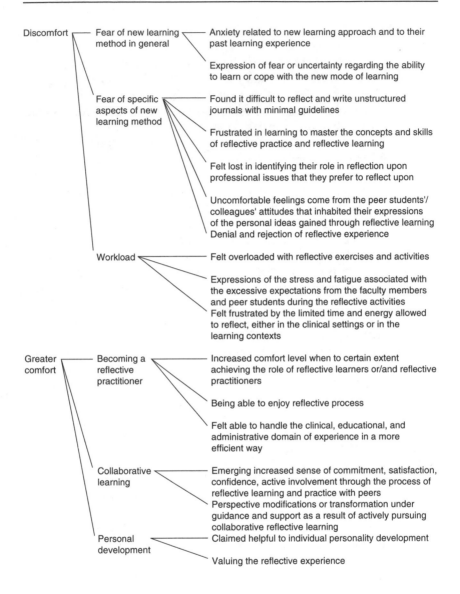

Fig. 10.1   Hierarchical categorisation of affective responses

Fear of new learning method

It is notable that prior to initial attempts to write reflective journal entries or engage in small group discussions of them, most participants felt anxious, frightened and insecure. The reason given was that this was a new learning mode quite different to previous passive learning styles. This is clearly illustrated by the following quotation from a student:

'In the past I was quite inflexible in my method of study. I only revised what the teachers said was important. Now I have to read books and find [relevant] material for myself. Of course they are different ... very different, so I am not able to cope with this [learning approach] ... I could not decide what was right or wrong, the feeling was so insecure. Through journal writing and sharing in the learning process, I found that writing papers is very difficult. Maybe I am still not familiar with the learning approach in tertiary education.'

Fear of specific aspects of new learning method

Students' anxiety was heightened by uncertainty over their ability to reflect and master reflective skills. The anxiety level was so intense that a student wrote:

'I was distressed with the feedback from the lecturer, I thought I was inadequate ... In fact I know that I could not reach the standard ... I do not have the ability to write the paper, and could not meet the requirement.'

Feelings of fear were common expressions since reflection required the individual to think critically about their daily practice. Although some students had little idea of the grounds for their feelings, it seems that they were afraid to reveal their inadequacy or incompetence at both a personal and the organisational level. A student verbalised her strain after reflecting upon daily practice:

'Sometimes it makes me worry, for example, I noticed I have done something in which I acted on impulse. In fact I should not have done it in this way, I will never do it again.'

Unsettling feelings were evident when the individual was unable to clarify and discriminate the conflicting values and associated behaviours upon reflection. A student was aware of her stress as she said, 'I was very frightened when my ideas were objected to by them [the peers]. I began to wonder if my idea was too innocent?' Boud, Cohen & Walker (1993) claimed more negative affective consequences would follow if the 'barriers' were not properly handled. This notion was supported by the view of another student who expressed her distress when she made this statement: 'I was even confused when I had more discussion.' In this circumstance, feelings of incompetence and inadequacy are inevitable.

The feeling of being abandoned was indicated when they felt they did not have clear enough guidelines on the tasks to be achieved. This feeling would subsequently impede the learning process. A student indicated her learning difficulties in relation to minimal guidelines when she commented:

> 'It would be better if we had been given some more guidelines ... I would perform better if I were given guidelines such as topic questions from the beginning ... We were worrying about our assignments when we submitted them because we did not know whether they were correctly done.'

Workload

Some students commented that they felt overwhelmed by excessive workloads or shortage of manpower and the pursuit of professional development. The issue of workload is particularly relevant to adult students for a demanding job and the pursuit of part-time study is never an easy combination. They were apprehensive that they could not perform as expected. The following description reflects their frustration at trying to practice reflection while facing imminent practical problems.

> '... Sometimes, frequently I could not reflect consciously because I had my own difficulties and pressure with my work. In fact people always have to make choices because of the limitation of time and energy.'

Increased comfort level

The above sections show that many students went through periods of quite intense discomfort and anxiety in their initial encounters with reflection on practice. However, as the course progressed the levels of anxiety diminished and more positive statements became apparent.

Positive feelings about becoming a reflective practitioner

The students' pattern of development was characterised by negative feelings of anxiety or fear on entering the reflective learning experience. Their feelings of 'uncertainty' diminished and they became more confident after they actively participated in the reflective activities. The following excerpt illustrates the student's positive feelings: 'When I became involved in [the reflective activities] I found that it was quite interesting.'

Collaborative learning

The support system, discussed later, helped the students become more confident in their ability to reflect upon their practice. Student peers acted as both confidants and role models in discussion sessions so more positive feelings developed and students gradually mastered reflective thinking. As this developed, it enhanced further participation in reflective practice. It was evident that the students showed appreciation in the arrangement of the reflective learning activities provided by the curriculum design as they asserted:

> 'I can come into contact with nurses from different hospitals and from different specialities ... I knew the perspectives of my peer students who are the nursing colleagues from different hospitals...'

In exploring the possibilities of modifying pre-dispositions in practice, they regarded positively the function of collaborative learning. One student stressed the role of peers in facilitating her reflective process:

> '... Later when I looked at the papers of others I found that my ideas were incorrect. In fact I could apply it to my working environment. I began to think in this way.'

Personal development

It is likely that when students commented that they had deliberately made efforts to be positive in relation to this learning process, they were able to turn the learning experience into an enlightening one. They consciously attempted to tolerate the uncomfortable feelings during the initial stage or before they were able to make further progress in reflection. The stimulating learning experience promoted the prospect of practising reflection. The narrative below shows a student who succeeded in overcoming the threats originating from the adverse feelings during initial reflective experience and was able to make prominent progress in reflective learning and practice.

The following series of quotations from one student illustrate the transition from discomfort with reflective thinking towards much more positive feelings. The quotations also hint at the role of fellow students and faculty members in easing this transition.

'I was afraid that I have nothing to report in the second discussion session...

I was very frightened when they [the peers] objected to my ideas. I began to think that my idea was too innocent? ... Then, I began to read books ... I was very happy because the person who wrote the foreword of the book shared similar ideas to mine ... They were the same as my idea...

... because we have sophisticated discussion, we can have a better understanding of the [professional] issue. Members from other groups raise questions during the discussion which can stimulate us to think more. Sometimes we are too focused on one part. These questions may arouse us to think from another perspective...

If I have arrived at an unfamiliar environment at work, I would reflect frequently. Later I would consider whether the procedure is appropriate and how to improve it...'

The support system

The peer group was shown to be a great support to the development of the reflective process. Although group discussion appeared to be threatening at the beginning, as the trusting atmosphere developed they felt support from others. To illustrate, one student stated:

'... At first when I discussed with my classmates, they were strongly against me ... As they did not have these ideas, they objected to mine. However, when we had second discussions on it, some of them began to remain neutral. When we discussed it further, some of them even agreed with me, so there was an integration of our thoughts ... Small group discussion helped me a lot. The other students are from different hospitals, different clinical units. Sometimes, they talked about their experiences which I have never heard before...'

The sharing of perspectives provides salient opportunities for learners to model necessary skills on reflection. Students shared their positive feelings with others about the success of putting theoretical knowledge into practice through peer dialogue interactions. With collaborative learning, the learners will feel more confident. Students are then empowered to take risks and question values and opinions held by those who practice their personal knowing.

Some students appreciated the presence of the faculty in the dialogues with their peers during the reflective learning experience. Students indicated the importance of trust building between the faculty and students in this study. The following quotation expresses this feeling:

> 'Of course, it's useless [to reflect alone] because I believed that I still cannot facilitate my self at this stage, I still need help, so I prefer discussion with a tutor. They can help us when there is need. I know that some tutors were very patient in explaining to the students.'

Discussion

The difficulties that students faced in adapting to the new method of teaching and learning is apparent from the quotations. For most of the students, their previous educational experiences could largely be summed up as didactic teaching and passive learning. Abandoning this mode, by having to take greater responsibility for their own learning, was obviously a quantum leap for the students.

What is particularly difficult about making the transition is that it is hard to give precise directions about what should be done and the final goal of reflective thinking and learning cannot be defined succinctly. Students who have grown used to receiving well-defined procedures and knowledge are faced with a journey entailing an ill-defined route towards an uncertain destination.

Conceptual change

Students have to make several associated conceptual changes in developing the ability to reflect upon their practice. Firstly, for our students at least, the approach to teaching was quite different from that which they had been accustomed to. In their previous experience the process of learning had largely been a passive role of absorbing transmitted material as directed by the teacher. The introduction to reflective thinking required students to adopt a more active approach to learning with the teacher taking a less directive role.

If the method for introducing reflection on practice involves reflective journal writing, as it normally does, then students have to adapt to a different form of writing. They have to unlearn practices which they will have been taught for most of their academic career. No doubt they have been taught that good academic writing cites academic authorities, is in the third person and the passive voice. In reports they are taught to focus upon outcomes.

If they are to become reflective writers they will have to learn that this alternative form of writing is characterised by the very qualities they have been taught to avoid. The substance of reflective writing is personal, and values, opinions and feelings are expressed. The struggle to achieve outcomes is often as valuable as the outcome itself.

Developing conceptions of knowledge

What is less readily apparent in the transcripts but is clearly implicit nevertheless, is the need for the students to develop appropriate conceptions of knowledge if they are to successfully engage in reflective thinking and judgement. This finding shows that the affective dimension is associated with any development through the seven stages of reflective judgement proposed by King & Kitchener (1994), reviewed in Chapter 1.

King & Kitchener's model of reflective judgement (1994) asserts that the ability to make reflective judgements about ill-structured problems is conditional upon reaching a sufficient development stage with respect to epistemological assumptions about knowledge (see Chapter 1). They argued that those in the lower developmental stages, in which knowledge is viewed as having a degree of certainty, would find it difficult to engage in reflective thinking.

The discomfort shown by students in attempting to employ reflective thinking and their reluctance to abandon the didactic teaching/passive learning view of education are indicative of pre-reflective thinking. The statements from students classified under the discomfort branch of the classification hierarchy are replete with terms such as 'right', 'wrong', 'correctly done', 'ideas were incorrect'. The information collected was insufficient to place students in a precise category of the reflective judgement model, but clearly students were at that time in one of the first three non-reflective levels because they saw knowledge as absolute.

The preference for a continuance of didactic teaching is

another indicator of their level. Where knowledge is viewed as a commodity with a high degree of certainty, a preference for didactic teaching makes a great deal of sense. The role of the teacher is that of the expert who can pass on a body of verified knowledge. The students see their role as absorbing it as well as possible.

The transcript material classified under the more positive branch shows evidence of students who have struggled to higher level conceptions of knowledge. It becomes apparent that students who have reached the higher levels see knowledge as something which is constructed. It was hard to make precise comparison with King & Kitchener's levels, particularly since their level definitions were given in terms of an individual. In their statements, which refer to knowledge being constructed, our students appeared to see it as a socially constructed phenomenon.

Assisting the change

There is a large body of research into changing student conceptions which shows how difficult the process is (e.g. Champagne, Gunstone & Klopfer, 1985). Strike and Posner (1985) characterise cognitive change in terms of advances, retreats and periods of indecision. As the project revealed, the literature suggests that students need to go through phases of disequilibrium and then re-conceptualisation.

From the field of science education, Champagne, Gunstone & Klopfer (1985) report changes in student conceptions of physics phenomena after several day-long sessions of ideational conflict but quotations from some of the students illustrate the demanding nature of the process. In a wider context, the pioneering work of Lewin (1952) on bringing about social change through group decision-making suggests a three-step procedure: unfreezing, moving and freezing of a level. Nussbaum & Novick (1982) and West (1988) suggest that, in an educational context, a similar three-phase process be required to bring about conceptual change. These are:

- A process for diagnosing existing conceptual frameworks and revealing them to the students.
- A period of disequilibrium and conceptual conflict which makes students dissatisfied with existing conceptions.
- A reconstruction or reforming phase in which a new conceptual framework is formed.

Chapters 4 to 9 have discussed at length the authors' own conclusions about helping students along this path. Many of the students started with a set of related beliefs about teaching, learning and knowledge. Most of their learning experiences had been as passive recipients of knowledge presented didactically by a teacher. The teacher or the education department defined the content of the syllabus so the students came to see knowledge as something decided by experts which they had to absorb and reproduce in examinations.

Developing them beyond this set of beliefs required more student-centred approaches to teaching and learning. Rather than sitting passively in class, they were active in constructing knowledge. Not all the information came from the teacher following a designated syllabus. Instead they were led to recognise that their own experiences were of value and it was legitimate for them to determine which areas of knowledge were valuable to them.

Care had to be taken in weaning students away from didactic types of teaching and learning, with which they were familiar, towards ones which placed greater responsibilities in their own hands. 'Dropping them in at the deep end' would no doubt have left many drowning. It was important to structure the teaching arrangements so that support came from both teachers and fellow students.

In terms of helping students to deal with the affective dimension, the resistance of learners to taking an active role in the acquisition of reflective skills needs to be addressed. It is essential to develop strategies to minimise the students' feeling of lack of guidance and support during the initial learning experience. There is little doubt that these learners' past learning experiences exert a great deal of influence on their dispositions towards personal and professional development. The role of the supportive teachers is to provide students opportunities to talk privately about their reflective experience. This assists the individual in rationalising the anxiety-filled situations. They will be more capable of confronting their tacit assumptions about teaching and learning and ready to make the paradigm shift towards reflecting upon practice.

In the transcripts, mention of group discussion often occurs in conjunction with evidence of belief that knowledge is constructed and thus a higher level of comfort in employing reflective thinking. We feel this conjunction strengthens our findings that group discussion is an important element in helping students develop critical thinking abilities. It seems to work towards both developing more appropriate conceptions of knowledge and a better understanding of the nature of reflective thinking and writing.

Chapter 11
Triggers for reflection

David Kember

Introduction

This is the second chapter in which the nature of reflection is
re-examined. In this chapter the emphasis is upon the starting
points or the triggers for reflection. What is it which stimulates professionals to reflect upon their action? In examining
our database we discovered that there were many ways in
which reflection had been triggered. These starting points
were structured into a hierarchical classification scheme.

Included within the scheme were the instances of reflection
following a hiatus or unusual case in professional practice.
We also, though, found many cases in which reflection had
been deliberately stimulated. These occurred both in
professional practice and in an academic context.

Examining the various ways in which reflection had been
triggered we came to a re-examination of the breadth of the
construct of reflection. The data suggested the value of a holistic view. This chapter seeks to provide a wider perspective.

In concert with one of the main themes of the integration
of theory and practice, there is a discussion of the ways in
which reflection is triggered in professional practice and in
arranged post-mortems, and in theory and clinical practice in
academic settings. Both contexts show that reflection can
follow a more difficult case in the clinical setting, or a
situation can be arranged to stimulate the reflective process.
Various strategies used in the case studies to arrange and
stimulate reflective thought are discussed. In examining these
cases we become involved in a discussion of the process of
reflective thinking as an individual and a group activity.
Taken together, the examination of the triggers for reflective
thinking shows that the breadth of the concept of reflection is
broader than that portrayed in some of the literature which
takes a compartmentalised view following from a particular
disciplinary tradition.

The analysis went through several stages. Initially the collected statements on reflection were examined for broad areas of significance. This chapter is concerned principally with triggers for reflection but does draw upon other broad categories as there were several other topics of interest which were conceptually related to this theme. The team then attempted to categorise the triggers for reflection. After two stages of refinement, the hierarchical scheme shown in Figure 11.1 was developed. The boundaries of the hierarchy were limited by the collected data-set. Had more data been available from practice or professional situations it would almost certainly have been possible to sub-divide the professional node into further sub-branches.

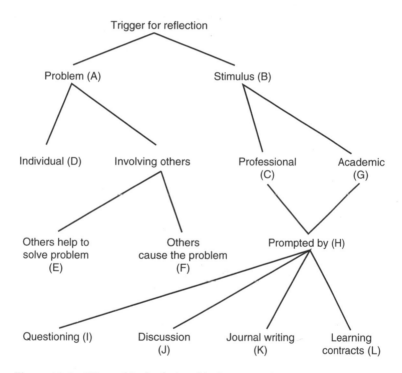

Figure 11.1   Hierarchical relationship between triggers

It should also be noted that, as with any classification system, it is often difficult to devise categories which are mutually exclusive. A common example for this study occurred over the academic/professional distinction. Cases which were not always clear cut in this respect were those involving professionals, who were also part-time students, reflecting upon their professional practice during a class session. Similar dichotomies arose with full-time students during their periods of professional practice.

Themes

Having developed the hierarchical classification scheme for triggers to reflection, it was found that several of the themes of interest which emerged from the original collection of statements about reflection could be exemplified through one or more of the categories in the hierarchy. These main themes are listed below.

(1) Reflection can occur through stimuli other than problems or disturbances to the normal routine. The stimuli may be encouraged or arranged.
(2) Reflection can be both an individual and a group activity. Group discussion can serve well as a spur to reflection.
(3) Reflection can and does take place in an academic environment. This includes the theory part of programmes and not just the professional practice component.
(4) The transcripts revealed several strategies, such as questioning, discussion and journal writing, for promoting fruitful reflection.
(5) Reflection is a broader concept than that portrayed in some literature on the topic, which tends to refer only to the context of professional practice.

The relationship between the themes and the trigger categories is shown in Figure 11.2. The themes are given in italics and their relationship to the trigger categories indicated by the boxes. To aid the reader in following the arrangement of the chapter, the themes have been numbered from 1 to 5 in the above list and on the diagram. Categories within the hierarchy which are discussed in the text have been lettered from A to K. Headings within this chapter are followed by a number or letter in parentheses to indicate which theme and/ or element of the trigger hierarchy is discussed.

The chapter will now illustrate the categories in the hierarchical classification system of the triggers for reflection through quotations which are typical of those in that category. At appropriate points in this exposition the five themes above will be addressed.

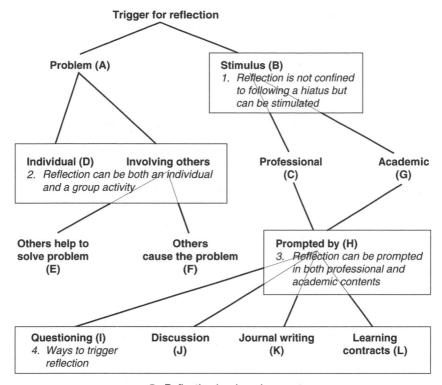

Figure 11.2   Themes and triggers

Reflection following a problem (A)

Schön (1983) believed that the thought processes underlying much of the routine work of professionals takes place almost unconsciously. In standard cases professionals display an almost unconscious routine which Schön calls *knowing-in-action*. *Reflection-in-action* is reserved for cases and situations which do not come within the normal routine.

> 'There is some puzzling, or troubling, or interesting phenomenon with which the individual is trying to deal. As he tries to make sense of it, he also reflects on the understandings which he surfaces, criticises, restructures and embodies in further action.'   (Schön, 1983, p. 50).

Atkins & Murphy (1993) reviewed work on the mechanism for reflection and concluded that most authors (Mezirow, 1981; Schön, 1983; Boud, Keogh & Walker,

1985; Powell, 1989) shared a common understanding. Their synthesised model consisted of three stages:

- awareness of uncomfortable feelings and thoughts
- critical analysis
- new perspective

The discomfort mentioned in the first point would occur when a practitioner was dealing with a typical ill-defined problem, of the sort which are faced in normal practice, but one in which standard ways of tackling the issue or normal frameworks for understanding the problem did not seem to apply. This would lead to a trigger point occurring with the realisation that knowledge possessed was insufficient to explain what was happening in a unique situation. This self-realisation brought on a sense of inner discomfort. Our data included the following examples which illustrate this position.

- 'If a duty can be carried out smoothly as a normal procedure, I rarely make reflection. But for some emergency cases such as bleeding, I have to consider immediately the way to help the patient especially when our unit has so many new instruments.'

- 'Of course I will make reflection after I do something wrong. Otherwise I am quite passive. Whether I will do reflection depends on the frequency of happening of the matter. If an experience happens frequently, it can't catch my attention.'

- 'If your work is always smooth, you will not think about the issue. For example, a patient asks me what kind of food he should avoid. If I don't know the answer, I'll reflect on the reason as it makes me feel embarrassed.'

Stimuli to reflection (B and 1)

The notion that reflection follows a hiatus, problem, or perturbation to routine practice is common within the literature on reflection based on the context of professional practice. However, in our data we also found considerable evidence of reflection triggered by stimuli or events which could not be viewed as problematic or unforeseen.

The term *stimulus* is used as the category label and encompasses a range of catalysts to reflective thinking. The situations include meetings, reading items, discussions and planned events. At times the stimulus resulted from a normal part of the daily timetable, in other situations the informants deliberately set out to arrange or plan situations and conditions which would stimulate reflective thinking.

The discussion on reflection in an academic context, which follows, contains many quotations illustrating reflection triggered by a stimulus. These occur in both the professional practice component of courses and the theory part. There are examples where the strategies for promoting reflection have been deliberately planned into the curriculum. There are also examples of students spontaneously reflecting following the discovery of stimulating material or ideas. The example below shows a student stimulated by a clever solution by a more experienced fellow student.

'I have seen an impressive case which was performed by a higher level student. It was also portable [X-ray] projection. We went to the ward. There was a patient who had a multiple fracture. The records showed that it was fractured. There was a crutch. The doctor required us to give him a lateral cervical. At that time, the crutch had covered it. The higher level student told the doctor but the doctor insisted. The higher level student did not use 90-degree view but used 70-degree view instead. I think the higher form students has reflected on his basic knowledge and made a modification.'

Stimuli in a professional context (C)

There was, though, substantial evidence that this category was not confined to the academic sector. There were examples of professionals being stimulated to reflect and of deliberately setting out to create conditions which would stimulate reflection. The first example refers to a clinician thinking about her normal practice in a different way.

'In the past if somebody asked me to set up instruments for occupational therapy, I would do it immediately. I would not consult anybody. Now, for the same case, I will ask for advice before I make any decision. I was quite confident and always thought I was the best. But now I realise that I can learn something in this way.'

The second example is a case where work practices have been re-planned so as to encourage reflection within a small team.

'I am always trying to improve the quality of clinical reasoning. But I must admit, there are times when the case demand on workload is high, so that even though I may prepare the things well, I have to do more evaluation on past clinical blocks. It is not that easy, because we don't have enough time for that. But now, because we have an education sub-committee, at least the six clinical educators will come together regularly. I think it is a good time to reflect and know what is the situation now. Then we come up with better ideas than the individual clinical educators might have.'

Reflection as an individual or a group activity (2)

In Schön's (1983) work the descriptions of reflective thinking mostly refer to the thought processes of individual professionals. Even when discussing the education of future professionals (Schön 1987), case studies can refer to the reflective thinking of individual students with guidance from a master practitioner. The idea of an individual reflecting on his or her own actions has sufficient currency that the term *self-reflection* is widely used. von Wright (1992, p. 61) defines self-reflection and points out its limitations.

'Self-reflection implies observing and putting an interpretation on one's own actions, for instance considering one's own intentions and motives as objects of thought. Here, one's knowledge of oneself is in principle as 'indirect' as that of another observer, and may be even less reliable – a person may not always be the best judge of his or her intentions ... when I reflect about my own intention, I step back, as it were, and *interpret* it, and this interpretation is fallible, like all interpretations.'

Habermas (1974, p. 29) also warns that there are dangers associated with solitary self-reflection.

'The self-reflection of a lone subject ... requires a quite paradoxical achievement: one part of the self must be split off from the other part in such a manner that the subject can be in a position to render aid to itself ... in the act of self-reflection the subject can deceive itself.'

The work of Habermas underpins the critical model of action research (Carr & Kemmis, 1986). The integral reflective process of this form of action research is normally regarded as a group process. It is suggested that group discourse provides a mechanism by which participants become aware of unconscious assumptions or false perspectives. Mezirow (1981; 1991) and Mezirow & Associates (1990) describe the outcome as a perspective transformation.

In our data we found evidence of reflection as both an individual experience and a group activity. Some seemed to seek solitude to quietly reflect upon their own activities. Others needed a stimulus from one or more colleagues for reflective thinking to occur.

Individual (D)

The individual reflectors often spoke of the need for quiet, relaxing conditions before they could reflect upon their activities. The hustle and bustle of the professional routine was mentioned as a constraint upon reflective thought. Those who felt they should reflect upon their practice, seemed to set aside time in a sanctuary for reflective thinking.

> 'My own setting is so busy that there is no time for me to sit back and concentrate on certain issues. My own working environment does not allow this. I do not have my own table and the station is crowded around with patients. So the only time for me to reflect is lunchtime and after work.'

Group solutions (E)

Some seemed to find individual reflection difficult and needed to share the process with another. They used others, often one other, as a sounding board for working through their thoughts.

> 'I need to share what I reflect with somebody. It doesn't matter who, maybe you, maybe my student, or maybe my husband or maybe a friend. With these, it strengthens my points and thinking, and because I know that it is my weakness to find a way to express it. So, it will lead me to a way of solving it. I would ask others or somebody who shares this feeling to help me to reflect.'

Others found that the different perspectives of others could lead to new insights.

'But during inter-group discussion, a classmate mentioned she once wanted to do [. . .] but it was not practical because paper was too expensive. I found out the solution immediately. This is a real example. We came from different hospitals and the examples made me think more.'

There were also numerous examples of the value of group discussion as a stimulus to reflection.

'In the first meeting I found that I could learn something when I tried to listen to others' ideas. For example, sharing our incidents. I gave my response and I experienced their feelings. I began to have the patience to listen to them. Then I analysed what they said and gradually I became very happy. Each member of the group was so open-minded. We affected each other and gave responses to other's opinions.

Others causing a problem (F)

As well as these examples of group reflection leading to fruitful outcomes, there were instances where the need for reflection resulted from the action of others. These examples were classified under the problem branch of the hierarchical tree because they were interpreted as reflection on problems caused by the actions of others.

'For example, you know your Head dislikes some things. You know how to do it the next time when you have tried it and displeased him. If your Head is an anxious person, you have no reason to do something which he hates. At first you did it and he abused you because you didn't know that. So you will never do it again.'

The example below is an interesting one of others creating a problem which can be solved through joint reflection.

'The problem that I constantly think about is about how I deal with my colleagues. I feel dissatisfied with their performance. However, in my position as a senior nurse with my nursing officer, what advice I have given them may not be accepted by them, even though I try to be more humble or friendly. So once I find the problems, I will give some suggestions first, but sometimes I think it is no use. I always reflect about these problems when I meet with my nurse officer. We always do the reflection together and try to find a better method to adjust our junior staff to do their performance better.'

Strategies for promoting reflection in an academic context (G and 3)

Much of the more recent literature on reflection has dealt with the concept in a professional situation. This is presumably because of the impact of Schön's work. Furthermore, a substantial part of the educational literature referring to reflection does so in the context of programmes with a professional orientation. More specifically, the term is most frequently found in connection with the professional practice component of such courses.

The wider sense of reflective thinking in the way in which Dewey (1933) used the term is still to be found. However, by comparison to the mountain of writing on reflection in a professional context, the molehill of work retaining the more holistic sense of reflection has become overshadowed.

Even though our wider study was of professional education courses, there were numerous examples of reflective thinking which were not in the practice context. The reason was that a key feature of each of the courses was that they attempted to encourage reflection during the theory part of courses – not just the practice component. The main rationale here is an attempt to bridge the theory/practice divide. Reflective practice has been touted as a way of bridging the gap (e.g. Clarke, 1986; Tichen & Binnie, 1992; Conway, 1994) confining it to the professional practice component will obviously not help in this respect.

In the case of post-registration or in-service courses, it is possible for students to reflect upon their current practice.

'Small group discussion helped me a lot. They [fellow students] are from different hospitals, different wards. Sometimes, they talked about their experiences which I have never heard before. For example, patients with kidney disease and those on TB drugs. They shared their experiences and practices. I can remind myself what to do when I face similar situations. Reflective learning is like a light bulb in my mind, it will switch on suddenly but I have never written it down, so I think I have not done it completely.'

The pre-registration or pre-service courses also attempted to stimulate reflection. This was seen as important so as to send out a reflective practitioner into the workplace. As the students did not have professional experience to draw upon the introduction to reflection upon clinical experience had to be structured into the programme.

'I always encourage the students to think over what sorts of things they have to do. Sometimes, I give them a diagnosis before I bring in the case. After they have a look at the case, I will then ask them what sorts of things they would like to perform before they go out to do it during the initial assessment. In this case, they have the time to think it over first. Especially for the earlier level students, because they always perform in a group, I feel it is the right time to bring in such case. But for high level students, I would let them do it in their own time.'

Prompting reflection in an academic context (H and 4)

The interviews and journals revealed a number of strategies which teachers or clinical educators used to stimulate students to reflect. Those which involved interaction with others were divided into two categories of either discussion sessions or the use of questioning techniques. The courses also featured the use of reflective journal writing as a stimulus to reflection.

Questioning (I)

Students could see the value of questioning and guidance.

'[...] really stimulated me to understand the [...] case more through her questioning. Actually, she let me think more about the theory behind the treatment. I found her guidance was useful, too.'

An interesting example below shows that the questions of the students can stimulate a clinical educator to reflect. In return the clinical educator uses questioning techniques to prompt student reflection.

'Students always ask you questions and ask you 'Why is it like that?' 'Why can't I do something like that?' With this kind of questioning, it will form some kind of stimulant. You will need to collect your knowledge and experience in order to analyse all these things. And after the evaluation, you need to give feedback or results back to the students. I think it is so important especially in this contemporary society. What is taught to the students may always change from what we have learnt before. So I need to adjust my experience and adjust my attitude, so that I will not be outdated. So I think it is quite important and useful for me. I will try to guide the students to use this kind of reflection process for them to learn. So I always use those stimulating questioning words like, why, what, which, how, in order to make them think.' (clinical educator)

However, not all questioning was conducive to reflection.

'When you are in the placement, there are some clinical instructors asking you some questions. In Year 1, they assume you don't know and you will ask them definitely. But if you are Year 2 and Year 3, although what they ask is called questions, and they will also encourage you to ask them back. Actually the feeling they give you and their attitudes show that they assume you must know it, or you have asked other staff in that hospital. They never think you will ask them questions back. There are many times that they will ask whether you have an opinion or whether you have anything to ask, you sure say no. There is another situation that if you see the clinical instructor is in hurry to have a meeting and he has many things to do, he will ask you whether you have something to ask. You don't want to hinder him doing his job and you say no.'

The questioning needed to be open-ended and stimulating. The manner of the questioner was also important. The student needs to feel safe and unthreatened for reflection to occur.

'I think it depends on the encouragement given by the people around you. For example, among all the place-ments, I reflected most in the [...] Hospital. It is because their seniors are very nice and they will encourage you all the time if you do well. They will not leave you in a room, of course you do your job by yourself, but they will see you regularly and ask about the progress. If they think you do quite well, they will encourage you. And the staff are rather nice. If you have anything you don't understand and ask, or if you have some new ideas and ask him if they work, they will love to discuss with you. I think it depends on the environment. If you ask me about the situation which

encourages me to do most in my three-year university life, I
guess it is a friendly and safe clinical situation.'

Discussion (J)

The questioning was normally on a one-to-one basis.
Stimulation for reflection also occurred through organised
group discussions. The way in which these are structured is
important as not every group discussion results in reflection
by any means.

'At first, none of us are familiar with the topic so we didn't
have any materials for reflection. After the discussion and
challenging by classmates we can discuss it further. Furthermore, there is a presentation again. There may be new
findings and we can also respond to another's challenge.
This three-stage method may help.'

Again the role and approach of the tutor is important.
Didactic approaches are unhelpful. Students need to be
challenged and stimulated to work things out for themselves,
but given enough support and guidance to do so.

'Although they didn't write up or they didn't verbally tell
us the definition, they really demonstrated that they have a
lot of knowledge on this. Like when we are sharing our
reflective journals during the class, I find that they can
easily link up some of the experiences with the theory and
they can easily add up a lot of points for us to think about
and to share and to stimulate us to continue the reflective
process. I think they demonstrated in the way of teaching
while concerning the definition or the knowledge of
reflection. I think they let us explore this rather than just
telling us, [...] means "blah blah blah".'

Chapter 9 dealt with the role of discussion in promoting
reflection in some detail.

Journal writing (K)

Journal writing was also successful as a spur to reflective
thinking. The nature of the writing process means that,
initially at least, it is an aid for self-reflective thinking. The
reflective writing can be revealed to others and used as the
material for group discussion. In this case journal writing

serves as both a tool for individual reflection and a source of stimuli for group reflection.

For more information about prompting reflective thinking through journal writing see Chapters 5 and 8.

Learning contracts (L)

The reflective journal is undoubtedly the most common written format used to encourage reflection. It was also found, though, that learning contracts could be an effective spur to reflection. The use of learning contracts is discussed in Chapter 5.

The breadth of reflection (5)

By examining accounts of what triggers reflection, this study came to the view that reflective thinking should be seen as a widespread phenomenon in the sense in which Dewey (1933) wrote about it. That it has had such an impact upon the professional practice literature has tended to relegate the application of the construct in a wider context to a place in the shade.

Of importance to the academic community, is the recognition that reflection can take place in an academic context and not just in an environment of professional practice. For programmes of professional practice, reflection can take place in both the university setting and the professional practice component of the course. Indeed, if reflection is seen as a bridge between theory and practice it is important that it is actively promoted within the theory parts of the course and not confined to the practice situation.

The study showed clearly that reflection is not confined to situations which are problematic. Rather, it can follow from a stimulus, and further this stimulus can be a deliberately arranged event. For the educator, this implies that programmes can be arranged so as to stimulate reflection.

Of the panoply of inter-laced themes which have emerged from the transcripts, the most important for the educator is perhaps that reflective thinking can be stimulated. It is not confined to professional practice and it does not just occur following a hiatus. Rather, it is possible to stimulate reflective thinking in both the theory and practice parts of professional development courses.

Examples here have shown students stimulated to reflective thinking through a variety of methods, which illustrates the contention that reflection can be both an individual and a group activity. Journal writing is commonly employed as a stimulus for individual reflection and journal entries can then serve as a spur for group discussion and reflection. Individuals and groups can be stimulated to reflect by probing, but sensitive, questioning from a tutor. The examples also show clearly the effectiveness of group discussion in triggering reflection.

Chapter 12
Reflections on reflection

David Kember

Introduction

In the many hours we have spent teaching the courses discussed in this book we have come to realise that students find reflection an elusive concept. This is hardly surprising since reflection is a highly abstract construct and many of our students have been much more familiar with dealing with concrete ideas. The situation is not helped by the fact that so few of the many who write about reflection have attempted to define or explain it. There appears to be an assumption that the reader will understand the concept – though if the reader is a student this is not a reasonable assumption. Where there are adequate explanations, they can often be inconsistent with those of writers from different discipline areas or epistemological backgrounds. We, therefore, feel obliged to draw together the insights we have gained into the nature of reflection in the course of this project.

Chapter 1 concluded with a tentative definition of reflection based upon attempts to draw together disparate strands of writing which have grown up within fairly discrete areas of the literature originating from different knowledge bases. In this final chapter this tentative definition is re-visited and developed further. We draw upon greater insights into the nature of reflection from our struggles to develop curricula which develop reflective thinking and help teach students to become reflective practitioners. The chapter also synthesises into the framework the conclusions reached in the previous two chapters.

As a starting point, the summary of characteristics of reflection – derived from the literature reviewed in Chapter 1 – is repeated here. In the remainder of the chapter this definition is expanded by adding elements from the previous two chapters, insights from teaching experiences and our

numerous discussions of the concept during our regular
reflective meetings.

- The subject matter of reflection is an ill-defined problem –
  the type of issues and cases dealt with in professional
  practice.
- The process of reflection may be triggered by an unusual
  case or can be deliberately stimulated.
- Reflection operates through a careful re-examination and
  evaluation of experience, beliefs and knowledge.
- Reflection most commonly involves looking back or
  reviewing past actions, though competent professionals
  can develop the ability to reflect while carrying out their
  practice.
- Reflection leads to new perspectives.
- Reflection operates at a number of levels, the highest level
  of critical reflection necessitates a change to deep-seated,
  and often unconscious, beliefs and leads to new belief
  structures.
- Reflective thinking ability is reached through a developmental process linked to developing appropriate conceptions of knowledge.

Affective dimension

Chapter 10 examined the affective dimension of reflective
thinking and particularly the difficult emotions many students encounter in trying to master the concept of reflecting
upon practice. The affective part of reflective thinking, in our
data, was most apparent in conjunction with students
undergoing conceptual changes necessary to engage in
reflective thinking and develop the ability to reflect upon
practice.

There was firstly a need to adapt from passive learning
methods they were used to and accept less directive teaching
and learning approaches. In learning to write reflective
journals the students had to unlearn conceptions of academic
writing and develop a more personal style. Finally most of
the students struggled with reflective judgement because their
conceptions of knowledge were not at the appropriate level
of King & Kitchener's hierarchy (1994). Many students
needed to move from positions in which knowledge was seen
as right or wrong, towards positions requiring interpretation
and the evaluation of evidence.

The process of developing beliefs about knowledge was

facilitated by exposing students to forms of teaching and learning other than the didactic content-led courses most of them had been used to. Instead they experienced process-oriented courses which were more student-centred. In these they learnt that their own experience and knowledge was valued. Group discussion helped to show that knowledge was socially constructed.

In making these conceptual changes it was common for students to initially feel considerable discomfort towards reflective thinking and the initial learning processes associated with it. As the arduous conceptual changes were made, the students' attitudes became much more positive. The difficult process of making these conceptual changes could be facilitated by support from student peer groups and tutors.

From our exploration of the affective dimension of reflection there are three further elements to add to the definition of reflection.

- There is an affective dimension associated with reflective thinking, which should not be underestimated.
- In making the conceptual changes necessary to develop reflective judgement, students commonly go through considerable discomfort until appropriate conceptions of knowledge are attained.
- Student peer groups and tutors can facilitate and support the student in undergoing these difficult conceptual changes needed for reflective judgement to develop.

Triggers for reflection

The previous chapter looked at the qualitative database to examine ways in which reflection was triggered. In the course of the analysis five themes emerged which are listed below for incorporation into the definition of reflection.

- Reflection can occur through stimuli other than problems or disturbances to the normal routine. The stimuli may be encouraged or arranged.
- Reflection can be both an individual and a group activity. Group discussion can serve well as a spur to reflection.
- Reflection can and does take place in an academic environment. This includes the theory part of programs and not just the professional practice component.
- Several strategies, such as questioning, discussion and journal writing, can be used for promoting fruitful reflection.

- Reflection is a broader concept than that portrayed in some literature on the topic, which tends to refer only to the context of professional practice.

Temporal dimension of reflection

In our regular reflective discussions during this project the concept of reflection was frequently discussed. Its presence as a component in the action research cycle caused us to consider the temporal aspects of reflection. The common portrayal of action research (e.g. Stenhouse, 1975; Carr & Kemmis,1986; Elliott, 1991; McKernan, 1991; McNiff, 1992) is as a cyclical process, with each cycle incorporating steps of planning, action, observation and reflection. There must be a delay in time between the action and reflection in one cycle and, if a series of cycles is followed, the action in the next.

Observing students also indicated a temporal nature to profound critical reflection. The most significant changes, such as the development of more sophisticated conceptions of knowledge took time. They occurred during the period of the course and could be marked by advances and retreats.

In Schön's (1983) categories of reflection, though, there is not always a delay between action and reflection. Indeed the types of reflection are distinguishable by the time frame over which they operate. Reflection-in-action occurs within the same time frame as the action. Reflection-on-action occurs afterwards. Our term of reflection-on-reflection-in-action implies a greater time delay again. If an arranged stimulus is the spur to engage in reflection there is necessarily a delay between the original act and the reflection upon it.

The temporal dimension of reflective thinking would also seem pertinent to the work of writers, such as Mezirow (e.g. 1991; Mezirow and Associates 1990) and van Manen (e.g. 1977), who distinguish their categories by the depth of reflective thinking or the extent to which perspectives are transformed. While the terminology varies somewhat, the writers agree that there is a level of critical reflection or perspective transformation which is more profound than standard reflection. Dewey (1933) saw critical reflective thinking involving a more considered and thorough examination of an issue.

Mezirow (1990; 1991) characterised the more profound level of reflection by a fundamental shift in underlying beliefs. Such major shifts in unconscious assumptions are widely seen as difficult and often painful processes. Perspective transformation and conceptual change are often characterised by advances and retreats. Deeper or more critical levels of reflection must inevitably, therefore, operate over an extended timeframe. Instant conversion surely occurs only in works of fiction. Reflection which follows action almost immediately is surely not critical reflection.

- Reflection-in-action implies that action and reflection are almost simultaneous.
- More critical reflection, involving perspective transformation, is likely to take some time so there will be a significant period between initial observations and final conclusions.

Teaching for reflection

We started chapter 1 by arguing that professionals need to become reflective practitioners because their practice entails dealing with messy problems. Developing a curriculum and a teaching approach to teach students reflective thinking and develop the capacity to reflect upon practice is itself a messy problem – a very 'wicked' problem.

Three main characteristics of messy problems were identified. The problems themselves need to be identified and it will be possible to envisage several issues. They will contain multiple dimensions, which will interact, so need to be tackled as an interacting system residing in the 'swampy lowland'. No ideal solution will be possible but reasonable positions which balance conflicting tensions should be sought. Developing a curriculum for reflective thinking contains each of these aspects of the ill-defined problem.

Chapters 3 to 7 dealt principally with a particular issue or design for developing reflective thinking. Though, it must be said that while the focus was upon one particular strategy, other elements of the situation were necessarily addressed within each of the sub-projects. Chapter 3 dealt with the action research approach used to implement, evaluate and refine the initiatives for reflective teaching and learning. Chapter 4 was concerned primarily with the integration of theory and practice. The next two chapters discussed the use of two strategies for promoting reflection, namely reflective journal writing and learning contracts. Chapter 7 reported on the use of written journal entries as a spur for small group tutorial discussion.

Part III, synthesised conclusions about teaching and curriculum designs from insights gained from the initiatives within individual courses, described in Part II. It is in this section of the book that we come to grips with the fact that the ill-defined problem of the reflective thinking curriculum has multiple conflicting elements which must be dealt with. We neither sought nor found an ideal solution but did arrive at some positions which benefited learning from adopting particular strategies while minimising conflicting tensions from other aspects of the teaching and learning system.

For example, Chapters 7 and 9 looked at the issue of disclosure in reflective writing. Free access to reflective journals, especially by the teacher, can inhibit students from revealing sensitive feelings or disclosing weaknesses, particularly if the disclosure is for assessment purposes. On the other hand, if the journal remains private there is no opportunity for the teacher to provide feedback to assist students to develop the capacity to write reflectively. As this feedback was found to be essential in developing reflective writing, we decided some level of disclosure was necessary. It was important, though, that before disclosure a position of trust was established between tutor and students and that the students accepted the need and the benefits of receiving feedback on their writing. At the early stages of the writing and commenting process, no assessment of writing should be attempted.

Another strategy coped with disclosure during small group tutorial discussion. Basing the discussion upon material within the journals proved to be a way to stimulate lively and profound interaction. The privacy concern was circumvented by establishing the ground-rule that each student was obliged to raise one issue each tutorial from the journal but beyond that reflections could remain private. However, we found in practice that the groups developed levels of rapport such that little was held back.

It is already clear that the issue of disclosure is inextricably inter-twined with the dilemma of assessment. Assessment of journal writing again tends to discourage open disclosure of difficulties and weaknesses as students are used to being awarded lower marks if they cannot do something. The form of writing all too easily ends up as a polished piece of traditional academic writing. If there is no assessment of writing, however, students do not see it as an essential part of the curriculum so do not take it seriously, or do not do it at all. One of the middle positions reached on the assessment issue was that of not assessing journal writing during the course but asking students to write an assessed final assignment developed from their formative journal writing.

There is no need to illustrate further the way we dealt with the messy curriculum design problems inherent in teaching reflective thinking and developing students' ability to reflect upon practice. The teaching strategies we developed and the positions we judged best, balanced the conflicting tensions have been described in detail in Parts II and III:

- When devising curricula and teaching strategies for reflective learning, it is necessary to view the teaching and learning environment as an ill-defined problem and seek positions which balance conflicting tensions.

What is worth re-iterating at this stage is the approach we found necessary to arrive at these compromise positions or most reasonable solutions to ill-defined problems. The cyclical approach of action research is ideal for introducing innovations into the swampy lowlands of the teaching and learning environment. It has a mechanism for trying out ideas, evaluating their effectiveness and further testing refined versions in subsequent cycles:

- The action research approach is ideal for introducing and refining teaching initiatives so as to arrive at these positions of balance.

The final point is to reiterate one of the themes which has run throughout the book. This concerns the integration of theory and practice. This has often been cited as a rationale for introducing students to the concept of reflective thinking. However, it is surprising how few professional courses themselves integrate theory and practice by developing students' skills in reflective judgement during the theory part of the course. We maintain that theory and practice will not be integrated unless this happens. Further, students will not be prepared for reflecting upon their practice during clinical or professional practice sessions unless they have developed the ability to make reflective judgements during the theory part:

- The theory parts of courses should address the issue of developing reflective judgement so that theory is integrated with practice and students are equipped for reflection upon practice during periods of professional practice.

Conclusion

To conclude the book, the elements of our explanation of reflection are gathered together and incorporated with the key themes on reflective teaching and learning.

- The subject matter of reflection is an ill-defined problem – the type of issues and cases dealt with in professional practice.
- In professional practice the process of reflection may be triggered by an unusual case or deliberate attempts to revisit past experiences.
- Reflection can occur through stimuli other than problems or disturbances to the normal routine. The stimuli may be encouraged or arranged.
- Reflection operates through a careful re-examination and evaluation of experience, beliefs and knowledge.
- Reflection most commonly involves looking back or reviewing past actions, though competent professionals can develop the ability to reflect while carrying out their practice.
- Reflection leads to new perspectives.
- Reflection operates at a number of levels, the highest level of critical reflection necessitates a change to deep-seated, and often unconscious, beliefs and leads to new belief structures.
- Reflection-in-action implies that action and reflection are almost simultaneous.
- More critical reflection, involving perspective transformation, is likely to take some time so there will be significant periods between initial observations and final conclusions.
- There is an affective dimension associated with reflective thinking which should not be underestimated.
- Reflective thinking ability is reached through a developmental process linked to developing appropriate conceptions of knowledge.
- In making the conceptual changes necessary to develop reflective judgement students commonly go through considerable discomfort until appropriate conceptions of knowledge are attained.
- Student peer groups and tutors can facilitate and support the student in undergoing these difficult conceptual changes needed for reflective judgement to develop.
- Reflection can be both an individual and a group activity. Group discussion can serve well as a spur to reflection.

- Reflection can and does take place in an academic environment. This includes the theory part of programmes and not just the professional practice component.
- Strategies, such as questioning, discussion and journal writing can be used to promote fruitful reflection.
- When devising curricula and teaching strategies for reflective learning, it is necessary to view the teaching and learning environment as an ill-defined problem and seek positions which balance conflicting tensions.
- The action research approach is ideal for introducing and refining teaching initiatives so as to arrive at these positions of balance.
- The theory parts of courses should address the issue of developing reflective judgement so that theory is integrated with practice and students are equipped for reflection upon practice during periods of professional practice.
- Reflection is a broader concept than that portrayed in some literature on the topic, which tends to refer only to the context of professional practice.

References

Anderson, G., Boud, D. & Sampson, J. (1996) *Learning Contracts. A Practical Guide*. Kogan Page, London.

Argyris, C., Putnam, R. & Smith, D. (1985) *Action Science*. Jossey-Bass, San Francisco.

Atkin, J.M. (1968) Behavioural objectives in curriculum design: A cautionary note. *The Science Teacher*, May.

Atkins, S. & Murphy, K. (1993) Reflection: A review of the literature. *Journal of Advanced Nursing*, **18**, 1188–92.

Baker, L. & Braun, A.L. (1984) Metacognitive skills and reading. In: *Handbook of Reading Research* (eds D. Pearson, M.L. Kamil, R. Barr & R. Mosenthal, 353–94, Longman, New York.

Bean, T.W. & Zulich, J. (1989) Using dialogue journals to foster reflective practice with pre-service, content-area teachers. *Teacher Education Quarterly*, **16** (1), 33–40.

Benner, P. (1984) *From Novice to Expert*. Addison-Wesley, Menlo Park.

Biggs, J.B. (1999) *Teaching for Quality Learning at University. What the Student Does*. Society for Research into Higher Education and Open University Press, Buckingham.

Boud, D. (1981) *Developing Autonomy in Learning*. Kogan Page, London.

Boud, D. (1985) Problem-based learning in perspective. In: *Problem-based Learning in Education for the Professions* (ed D. Boud). Higher Education Research and Development Society of Australasia, Sydney.

Boud, D., Cohen, R. & Walker, D. (1993) *Using Experience for Learning*. Open University Press, Bristol.

Boud, D., Keogh, R. & Walker, D. (1985) *Reflection: Turning Experience into Learning*. Kogan Page, London.

Boud, D. & Walker, D. (1991) *Experience and Learning: Reflection at Work*. Deakin University, Geelong.

Boud, D. & Walker, D. (1993) Barriers to reflection on experience. In: Using Experience for Learning (eds D. Boud, R. Cohen & D. Walker). Open University Press, Bristol.

Boud, D. & Walker, D. (1998) Promoting reflection in professional courses: The challenge of context. *Studies in Higher Education*, **23**(2), 191–206.

Boyd, E.M. & Fales, A.W. (1983) Reflective learning: Key to learning from experience. *Journal of Humanistic Psychology*, **23**(2), 99–117.

Brookfield, S. (1993) Breaking the code: Engaging practitioners in critical analysis of adult education literature. *Studies in the Education of Adults*, **25**(1), 64–91.

Cameron, B.L. & Mitchell, A.M. (1993) Reflective peer journals: Developing authentic nurses. *Journal of Advanced Nursing*, **18**, 290–97.

Carper, B. (1978) Fundamental ways of knowing in nursing. *Advances in Nursing Science*, **1**(1), 13–23.

Carr, W. & Kemmis, S. (1986) *Becoming critical: Education, Knowledge and Action research*. Falmer Press, Sussex.

Champagne, A.B., Gunstone, R.F. & Klopfer, L.E. (1985) Effecting change in cognitive structures among physics students. In: *Cognitive structures and conceptual change* (eds L.H.T. West & A.L. Pines). Academic Press, New York.

Clarke, M. (1986) Action and reflection: Practice and theory in nursing. *Journal of Advanced Nursing*, **11**, 3–11.

Conway, J. (1994) Reflection, the art and science of nursing theory-practice gap. *British Journal of Nursing*, **3**(3), 164–72.

Denzin, N. (1970) *The Research Act in Sociology*, Butterworths, London.

Dewey, J. (1933) *How we Think: a Restatement of the Relation of Reflective Thinking to the Educative Process*. Heath, Boston: D.C.

Elliott, J. (1991) *Action Research for Educational Change*. Open University Press, Milton Keynes.

Eraut, M. (1985) Knowledge creation and knowledge use in professional contexts. *Studies in Higher Education*, **10**(2), 117–33.

Fish, D., Twinn, S., & Purr, B. (1990) *How to enable Learning through Professional Practice: a Cross-profession Investigation of the Supervision or pre-service Practice. A pilot study*. Report no. 1, West London Institute of Higher Education, London.

Garman, N.B. (1986) Reflection, The heart of clinical supervision. A modern rationale for professional practice. *Journal of Curriculum and Supervision*, **2**(1), 1–24.

Glaser, B.G. & Strauss, A.L. (1967) *The Discovery of Grounded Theory*. Aldine, Chicago.

Greenwood, J. (1998) The role of reflection in single and double loop learning. *Journal of Advanced Learning*, **27**(5), 1048–53.

Habermas, J. (1970) Towards a theory of communicative competence, *Inquiry*, **13**.

Habermas, J. (1972) *Knowledge and Human Interests*, (tr. J.J. Shapiro). Heinemann, London.

Habermas, J. (1974) *Theory and Practice*(tr. J. Viertel). Heinemann, London.

Habeshaw, S., Habeshaw, T. & Gibbs, G. (1984) *53 Interesting Things to do in your Seminars and Tutorials*. Technical and Educational Services, Bristol.

Hahnemann, B.K. (1986) Journal writing: a key to promoting critical thinking in nursing students. *Journal of Nursing Education*, **25**(5), 213–15.

Holter, I.M. & Schwartz-Barcott, D. (1993) Action research: what is it? How has it been used and how can it be used in nursing? *Journal of Advanced Nursing*, **18**, 298–304.

Jaques, D. (1991) *Learning in Groups*. Kogan Page, London.

Jarvis, P. (1987) *Adult Learning in the Social Context*. Croom Helm, London.

Jarvis, P. (1992) *Paradoxes of Learning: On becoming an Individual in Society*. Jossey-Bass, San Francisco.

Jarvis, P. (1995) *Adult and Continuing Education: Theory and Practice*, 2nd edition, Routledge, London.

Jones, A., Yeung, E. & Webb, C. (1998) Tripartite involvement in health care clinical education. *Journal of Allied Health*, **27**, 97–102.

Johns, C. (1995a) *The value of reflective practice for nursing*, **4**(1), Jan. 1995, 13–23.

Johns, C. (1995b) Framing learning through reflection within Carper's fundamental ways of knowing in nursing. *Journal of Advanced Nursing*, **22**, 226–34.

Johns, C. (1996a) *Visualizing caring in practice through guided reflection*, **24**(6), 1135–43.

Johns, C. (1996b) *Using a reflective model of nursing and guided reflection*, **11**(2), 34–38.

Kember, D. (2000) *Action Learning and Action Research: Improving the Quality of Teaching and Learning*. Kogan Page, London.

Kember, D. & Gow, L. (1992) Action research as a form of staff development in higher education. *Higher Education*, **23**(3), 297–310.

Kember, D., Charlesworth, M., Davies, H., McKay, J. & Stott, V. (1997) Evaluating the effectiveness of educational innovations: Using the Study Process Questionnaire to show that meaningful learning occurs. *Studies in Educational Evaluation*, **23**(2), 141–57.

Kember, D., Jones, A., Loke, A., McKay, J., Sinclair, K., Tse, H., Webb, C., Wong, F., Wong, M. & Yeung, E. (1999) Determining the level of reflective thinking from students' written journals using a coding scheme based on the work of Mezirow. *International Journal of Lifelong Education*, **18**(1), 18–30.

Kember, D. & Kelly, M. (1993) *Improving Teaching through Action Research*. Green Guide no. 14. HERDSA, New South Wales.

Kember, D. & McKay, J. (1996) Action research into the quality of student learning: A paradigm for faculty development. *Journal of Higher Education*, **67**(5), 528–54.

Kemmis, S. & McTaggart, R. (1982) *The Action Research Planner*, 3rd edn. Deakin University, Geelong.

King, P.M. & Kitchener, K.S. (1994) *Developing Reflective Judgement: Understanding and Promoting Intellectual Growth and critical Thinking in Adolescents and Adults*. Jossey-Bass, San Francisco.

Knowles, M.S. (1983) Applications in continuing education for the health professions. *Andragogy in action, MOBIUS*, **5**(2), 80–100.

Kolb, D. (1984) *Experiential Learning*. Prentice Hall, Englewood Cliffs, NJ.

Leino-Kilpi, H. (1990) Self-reflection in nursing teacher education. *Journal of Advanced Nursing*, **15**, 192–5.

Lewin, K. (1952) Group decision and social change. In: *Readings in Social Psychology* (eds G.E. Swanson, T.M. Newcomb & F.E. Hartley. Holt, New York.

Marton, F. (1981) Phenomenography – describing conceptions of the world around us. *Instructional Science*, **10**, 177–200.

Marton, F. (1986) Some reflections on the improvement of learning. In: *Student Learning: Research into Practice*, (ed. J.A. Bowden). Melbourne University, Melbourne.

Marton, F. & Säljö, R. (1976) On qualitative differences in learning, outcome and process I. *British Journal of Educational Psychology*, **46**, 4–11.

McCaugherty, D. (1991) The theory-practice gap in nurse education: Its causes and possible solutions. *Journal of Advanced Nursing*, **16**, 385–97.

McCaugherty, D. (1991a) The use of a teaching model to promote reflection and the experiential integration of theory and practice in first year student nurses: an action research study, *Journal of Advanced Nursing*, **16**, 534–43.

McKernan, J. (1991) *Curriculum Action Research*. Kogan Page, London.

McNiff, J. (1992) *Action Research: Principles and Practice*. Routledge, London.

Meyer, J.E. (1993) New paradigm research in practice: the trials and tribulations of action research. *Journal of Advanced Nursing*, **18**, 1066–72.

Mezirow, J. (1977) Perspective transformation. *Studies in Adult Education*, **9**(2), 153–64.

Mezirow, J. (1981) A critical theory of adult learning and education. *Adult Education*, **32**(1), 3–24.

Mezirow, J. (1985) A critical theory of self-directed learning. In: *Self-directed Learning: from Theory to Practice*, (ed. S. Brookfield), pp. 17–30. Jossey-Bass, San Francisco.

Mezirow, J. (1991) *Transformative Dimensions of Adult Learning*. Jossey-Bass, San Francisco.

Mezirow, J. (1992) Transformation theory: Critique and confusion. *Adult Education Quarterly*, **42**(4), 250–52.

Mezirow, J. (1998) On critical reflection. *Adult Education Quarterly*, **48**(3), 185–98.

Mezirow, J. & Associates (1990) *Fostering Critical Reflection in*

Adulthood. Guide to Transformative and emancipatory Learning. Jossey-Bass, San Francisco.

Neville, S. & Crossley, L. (1993) Clinical education: Perceptions of a clinical tutor's role. *Physiotherapy*, **79**(7), 459–64.

Nussbaum, J. & Novick, S. (1982) Alternative frameworks, conceptual conflict and accomodation: Toward a principal teaching strategy. *Instructional Science*, **11**, 183–200.

Owens, R. (1982) Methodological rigor in naturalistic inquiry: some issues and answers. *Educational Administration Quarterly*, **18**(2), 1–21.

Parsons, J.E. & Durst, D. (1992) Learning contracts: misunderstood and undertutilized. *The Clinical Supervisor*, **10**(1), 145–56.

Perry, W.G. (1970) *Forms of intellectual and ethical development in the college years*. Holt, Rinehart and Winston, New York.

Perry, W.G. (1988) Different Worlds in the same classroom. In: *Improving Learning*, (ed. P. Ramsden). Kogan Page, London.

Powell, J.H. (1989) The reflective practitioner in nursing. *Journal of Advanced Nursing*, **14**, 824–32.

Ramsden, P. (1992) *Learning to teach in Higher Education*. Kogan Page, London.

Rapoport, R.N. (1970) Three dilemmas in action research. *Human Relations*, **23**(6), 499–513.

Rice, A.K. (1971) *Learning for Leadership, interpersonal and inter-group Relations*. Tavistock Publications, London.

Richards, T.J. & Richards, L. (1991) The NUD•IST qualitative data analysis system. *Qualitative Sociology*, **14**(4), 307–24.

Richardson, G. & Maltby, H. (1995) Reflection-on-practice: enhancing student learning. *Journal of Advanced Nursing*, **22**(2), 235–42.

Saylor, C.R. (1990) Reflection and professional education: Art, science, and competency. *Nurse Educator*, **15**, 8–11.

Schartz, M. (1993) Researching while teaching: promoting reflective professionality in higher education. *Educational action research*, **1**(1), 111–34.

Schön, D.A. (1983) *The reflective Practitioner: how Professionals think in Action*. Basic Books, New York.

Schön, D.A. (1987) *Educating the Reflective Practitioner*. Jossey-Bass, San Francisco.

Snowball, J., Ross, K., & Murphy, K. (1994) Illuminating dissertation supervision through reflection. *Journal of Advanced Nursing*, **19**, 1234–40.

Sparks-Langer, G.M. Simmons, J.M. & Pasch, M. (1990) Reflective pedagogical thinking: How can we promote it and measure it? *Journal of Teacher Education*, **41**(4), 23–32.

Stenhouse, L. (1975) *An Introduction to Curriculum Research and Development*. Heinemann Education, London.

Stephenson, J. & Laycock, M. (1993) *Using Learning Contracts in Higher Education*, pp. 57–62. Kogan Page, London.

Strike, K.A. & Posner, G.J. (1985) A conceptual change view of learning and understanding. In: *Cognitive Structure and Conceptual Change*, (eds L.H.T. West & A.L. Pines). Academic Press, New York.

Tichen, A. & Binnie, A. (1992) What am I meant to be doing? Putting practice into theory and back again in new nursing roles. *Journal of Advanced Nursing*, **18**, 1054–65.

Tripp, D.H. (1990) Socially critical action research. *Theory into practice*, **24**(3), 158–73.

van-Manen, M. (1977) Linking ways of knowing with ways of being practical. *Curriculum Inquiry*, **6**(3), 205–27.

von Wright, J. (1992) Reflections on reflection. *Learning and Instruction*, **2**, 59–68.

Wagenaar, T.C. (1984) Using student journals in sociology courses. *Teaching Sociology*, **11**(4), 419–37.

West, L. (1998) Implications of recent research for improving secondary school science learning. In: *Improving Learning: new perspectives*, (ed P. Ramsden). Kogan Page, London.

Wong, F.K.Y., Kember, D., Chung, L.Y.F. & Yan, L. (1995) Assessing the level of reflection from reflective journals. *Journal of Advanced Nursing*, **22**, 48–57.

Yinger, R.J. & Clark, C.M. (1981) *Reflective journal writing: theory and practice*, Occasional Paper, no. 50, Institute for Research on Teaching, Michigan State University.

Zander, A. (1979) The psychology of group process. *Annual Reviews of Psychology*, **30**, 417–51.

Zuber-Skerrit, O. (1992) *Action Research in Higher Education: Examples and Reflections*. Kogan Page, London.

Index